Animal Models and Experimental Research in Medicine

Edited by Mahmut Karapehlivan, Volkan Gelen and Abdulsamed Kükürt

Published in London, United Kingdom

Animal Models and Experimental Research in Medicine
http://dx.doi.org/10.5772/intechopen.100993
Edited by Mahmut Karapehlivan, Volkan Gelen and Abdulsamed Kükürt

Contributors
Emina Dervišević, Muhamed Katica, Adis Salihbegović, Lejla Dervišević, Zurifa Ajanović, Sabaheta Hasić, Lourdes Rodríguez-Fragoso, Anahi Rodríguez-López, Janet Sánchez-Quevedo, Lianhua Bai, Deyu Hu, Min Yan, Zhenyu Wu, Jiejuan Lai, Hongyu Zhang, Sijin Li, Leida Zhang, Uloma B. Elvis-Offiah, Success Isuman, Marvelous Johnson, Vivian Ikeh, Sandra Agbontaen, Abdulsamed Kükürt, Mahmut Karapehlivan, Volkan Gelen, Takahiko Aoki, Pilar Rojas, Ana I. Ramírez, Rosa de Hoz, Manuel Cadena, Juan J. Salazar, Elena Salobrar-Garcia, Inés López-Cuenca, José A. Fernández-Albarral, José M. Ramírez, Lidia Sanchez-Puebla, José Antonio Matamoros, Hidetoshi Masumoto, Hiroaki Osada, Kozue Murata, Atanas Arnaudov, Desisslava Arnaudova, Diego Torrecillas Paula Lico, Manoj Shah

First published in London, United Kingdom, 2023 by IntechOpen
IntechOpen is the global imprint of INTECHOPEN LIMITED, registered in England and Wales, registration number: 11086078, 5 Princes Gate Court, London, SW7 2QJ, United Kingdom

British Library Cataloguing-in-Publication Data
A catalogue record for this book is available from the British Library

Additional hard and PDF copies can be obtained from orders@intechopen.com

Animal Models and Experimental Research in Medicine
Edited by Mahmut Karapehlivan, Volkan Gelen and Abdulsamed Kükürt
p. cm.
Print ISBN 978-1-80356-653-5
Online ISBN 978-1-80356-654-2
eBook (PDF) ISBN 978-1-80356-655-9

For EU product safety concerns:
IN TECH d.o.o., Prolaz Marije Krucifikse Kozulić 3, 51000 Rijeka, Croatia,
info@intechopen.com or visit our website at intechopen.com.

Meet the editors

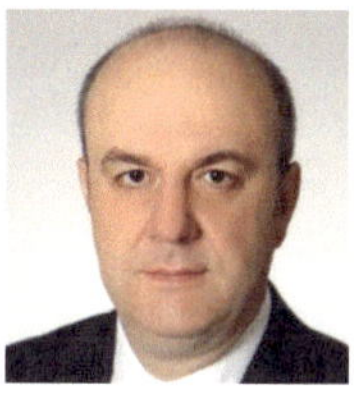

Prof. Dr. Mahmut Karapehlivan graduated from the Faculty of Veterinary Medicine, Kafkas University, Turkey, in 1995. That same year, he began his academic career at the same university as a research assistant in the Department of Biochemistry. In 2003, he completed his Ph.D. in Biochemistry at the Institute of Health Sciences, Kafkas University. In 2009, he became an Associate Professor of Biochemistry. He is currently a professor doctor in the Medical Faculty, Department of Medical Biochemistry, Kafkas University. He has published seventy journal papers, seven book chapters, and seventy-three conference presentations. Dr. Karapehlivan has also been the principal investigator or co-investigator in twenty-two research projects.

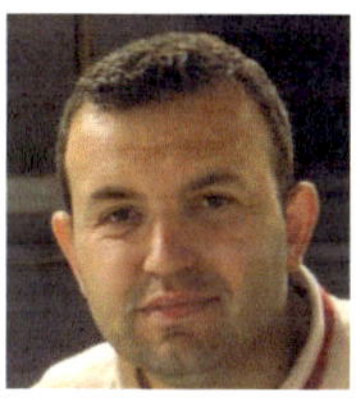

Dr. Abdulsamed Kükürt graduated from Uludağ University, Turkey. In 2019, he obtained a Ph.D. in Biochemistry from the Institute of Health Sciences, Kafkas University, Turkey, where he is currently an assistant professor in the Department of Biochemistry. He has published twenty-nine research articles in academic journals, fourteen book chapters, and thirty-seven papers. Dr. Kükürt has participated in ten academic projects and is a reviewer for many academic journals.

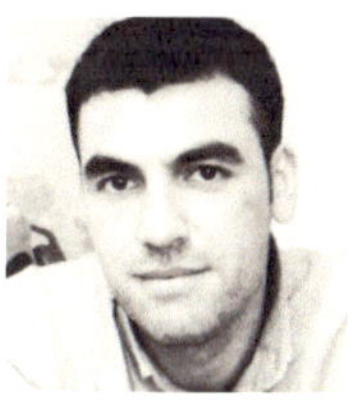

Dr. Volkan Gelen is a physiology specialist who received his veterinary degree from Kafkas University, Turkey, in 2011. From 2011 to 2015, he worked as an assistant in the Department of Physiology, Faculty of Veterinary Medicine, Atatürk University, Turkey. In 2016, he joined Kafkas University as an assistant professor where he has been engaged in various academic activities. Dr. Gelen has sixty journal articles and twenty poster presentations to his credit. His research interests include physiology, the endocrine system, cancer, diabetes, cardiovascular diseases, and isolated organ bath system studies.

Contents

Preface

Animal models and experimental research in medicine involve the use of animals to learn more about diseases and treatments in humans. Animal models are used to understand physiological, biochemical, and pathological mechanisms of cells, tissues, organs, and systems to elucidate inter-system relations and develop new diagnostic methods for diseases or functional disorders as well as new strategies for their treatment. Research may involve testing the effects of new drugs on animal models or studying the effects of environmental factors on the progression of diseases. Animal models are also used to gain insights into the behavior of disease processes and to develop new diagnostic tools and treatments. Evaluation of some biomarkers and even researching and finding new biomarkers to diagnose prognosis and treatment of diseases that are seen frequently will both help in the treatment of diseases and shorten this process considerably.

Animal Models and Experimental Research in Medicine contains chapters authored by international researchers that address experimental models of amyotrophic lateral sclerosis, hepatotoxicity, liver fibrosis/cirrhosis, visceral hyperalgesia, and female reproduction, as well as some fish studies and cardiovascular research in large animal models. Overall, this book offers essential information that will be helpful to researchers and scientists in medicine, biology, veterinary medicine, and other related fields who are interested in learning more about animal models and experimental research in medicine as well as ideas that will contribute to future research. It is a useful resource for medical professionals, students, and educators who are looking to better understand how animal models can be used to study and treat diseases.

Mahmut Karapehlivan
Faculty of Medicine,
Department of Biochemistry,
Kafkas University,
Kars, Turkey

Abdulsamed Kükürt
Faculty of Veterinary Medicine,
Department of Biochemistry,
Kafkas University,
Kars, Turkey

Volkan Gelen
Faculty of Veterinary Medicine,
Department of Physiology,
Kafkas University,
Kars, Turkey

Section 1

Animal Models in Various Diseases

Chapter 1

Impact of Temperature on Morphological Characteristics of Erythrocytes and Heart Weight: Experimental Study on Wistar Rats

Emina Dervišević, Sabaheta Hasić, Lejla Dervišević, Zurifa Ajanović, Muhamed Katica and Adis Salihbegović

Abstract

The aim was to find what happens to heart weight and forms of erythrocytes antemortemly and postmortemly as a result of exposure to high water temperature. Total of 40 adult Wistar rats is divided into three groups, depending on water temperature exposure of 37°C (KG, n = 8), 41°C (G41, n = 16), and 44°C (G44, n = 16). Depending on the length of time of exposure to water, temperatures of 41 and 44°C are further divided into G41-AM, G41-PM, G44-AM, and G44-PM. The anesthetized rats were exposed to preheated water using the water bath. May-Grünwald-Giemsa coloring technique was applied to blood samples. Light microscopy was performed to detect poikilocytes. Heart weight was measured after dissection with a scale. A statistically significant difference in heart weight was found in the experimental groups ($p = 0.024$). The lowest value was observed in KG37 and was 0.99 ± 0.11 g, and the highest values were found in rats of the G41-PM group, with a mean value of 1.26 ± 0.26 g. There is a statistically significant difference between the experimental groups in forms of poikilocytes.

Keywords: poikilocytosis, antemortem, postmortem, rats, heat, heart

1. Introduction

1.1 Body temperature – values, fluctuations, and regulation

The physiological range of human body temperature is 36.8 ± 0.3°C [1]. During physical activity, body temperature can rise from 38 to 40°C, and exposure to extremely low ambient temperatures can lead to a decrease in body temperature to 35°C [2]. In clinical thermometry, the mean physiological oral temperature of 36.8 ± 0.9°C correlates with the end product of the energy of all enzymatic reactions. Metabolism, through the sum of all the body's cellular reactions, is usually measured as the amount of oxygen consumed. The standardized estimate of metabolism is the basal rate of metabolism, which depends on the activity of these physiological processes to maintain euthermia [3]. The physiological body temperature of the human body core is about 37°C and is controlled in a narrow range (33.2–38.2°C), and is further narrowed if oral measurements are neglected in favor of rectal, tympanic, or axillary measurements [4]. Abnormal deviations of the core temperature of even a few degrees will trigger the body's thermoregulatory mechanisms, and changes in temperature outside the physiological range can prove fatal. Measured body temperature above 42°C leads to cytotoxicity with protein denaturation and impaired deoxyribonucleic acid (DNA) synthesis [5], resulting in organ failure and neuronal damage. If body temperature falls below 27°C (hypothermia), associated neuromuscular, cardiovascular, hematological, and respiratory changes may prove equally fatal [6]. The core temperature is maintained in the range of +/ 6°C in the environment from 10–55°C, while the skin temperature varies depending on the environment. The temperature measured orally is from 36.5 to 37°C, while the rectal temperature is 0.5°C higher [7]. In humans, body temperature varies by about 1°C during the day, with a gradual increase during wakefulness and a decrease during sleep [8]. Daily fluctuations in body temperature are a strong effect of circadian rhythms [9] associated with a number of physiological functions, such as metabolism and sleep [10, 11]. Evidence in humans and rats shows that circadian temperature rhythm is controlled separately from locomotor activity rhythms [12]. The amount of core temperature formation depends on the intensity of metabolism, and it depends on basal metabolism, muscle activity, thyroxine, adrenaline, noradrenaline, sympathetic nervous system activity, cell temperature, and digestive system activity. Heat release depends on the rate of conduction to the skin surface and the rate of heat transfer from the skin to the environment. The skin and subcutaneous tissue participate in the thermal insulation of the body. Blood vessels can regulate heat transfer by constriction and dilatation [13]. Body temperature varies depending on where it is measured. In thermoregulatory research, it is common for the body to be divided into two sections—the outer core, which includes the skin and which mainly varies in temperature with the environment, and the inner core, which includes the central and peripheral nervous system and has a relatively stable temperature [13, 14]. The preoptic area of the anterior hypothalamus plays a major role in the regulation of body temperature [15]. Most nerves are more sensitive to heat than to cold. Heating these areas of the brain increases the body's sweating, and cooling interrupts any mechanism of heat loss. There are many more receptors on the periphery to register cold than heat and all act on the hypothalamus [16]. Heat receptors also exist in deep tissues and are exposed to body core temperatures. On both sides of the posterior hypothalamus at the level of the mammary corpuscles is the posterior hypothalamic region that integrates central and peripheral thermal sensations. The role in the regulation of body temperature is mediated by sweat glands that have cholinergic innervation (acetylcholine), and to some extent, they can be stimulated by adrenaline and noradrenaline, secrete primary secretion, which is a product of epithelial cells, depending on the intensity of sweating [17]. With poor sweating, the secretion takes more time to pass through the canals, and consequently, more sodium and chlorine ions are reabsorbed, and potassium, urea, and lactic acid ions are concentrated. The process of acclimatization is associated with the reduction of sodium and chlorine ions in sweat, which improves the preservation of body electrolytes [18]. The nervous system acts as a biological thermostat for heating and cooling inside the animal's body. Because animals use resources, such as energy, water, and oxygen, for thermoregulation, the nervous system monitors the abundance of these resources and adjusts thermoregulatory mechanisms accordingly. Hunger, dehydration, or hypoxemia alter the activity of temperature-sensitive neurons in the preoptic region of the hypothalamus. Other regions of the brain work together with the hypothalamus on the adaptability of thermoregulation. For example, the amygdala is likely to inhibit neurons in the preoptic area, overriding thermoregulation when there is a risk of hypothermia or overheating. Moreover, the hippocampus allows the animal to remember microcells that allow safe and efficient thermoregulation [19].

1.2 The body's response to hyperthermia

Hyperthermia is a condition of elevated body temperature, above the upper physiological limit [19, 20]. When the body is exposed to high temperatures, the secretion of interleukins 1 and 6 (IL-1 and IL-6) and tumor necrosis factor (TNF) alpha from excited immune cells, which act on thermoregulatory centers and consequently lead to setting the center to a higher temperature [20]. In the body's response to hyperthermia, it is important to distinguish between endogenous and exogenous hyperthermia. Exogenous hyperthermia occurs when the influx of heat from the external environment increases significantly, such as in tropical areas, in small enclosed spaces that do not have adequate insulation and airflow with artificial increase in air temperature, in the bathroom during bathing, in saunas, and in Turkish baths. The fastest exogenous hyperthermia develops when there is a combination of increased heat influx from the outside with difficulty in heat transfer. Under these conditions, heat transfer mechanisms, despite maximum activation, do not remove heat from the outside, and body temperature begins to rise. Thermoregulation is actively aimed at raising the temperature by the process of overheating, all with the aim of faster heat transfer. In the 1990s, science showed that hyperthermia was teratogenic to both humans and animals. The state of hyperthermia can be the result of two processes. One is impaired production and release of heat, conditionally speaking the relationship between body temperature and ambient temperature, and the other is the setting of the thermoregulatory center to a higher level [21]. When there is an increased ambient temperature, the body temperature level rises slightly to the newly set temperature and hyperthermia occurs. Temperature rise occurs due to reduced temperature release and increased thermogenesis. High-energy consumption is required to raise the temperature, so a feeling of exhaustion may be present. When the body temperature equalizes that of the thermoregulatory center, thermogenesis ceases (if pyrogen secretion has ceased). After that, the set temperature of the thermoregulatory center returns to a lower value and there is a gradual decrease in body temperature due to reduced thermogenesis and increased heat release. Infectious diseases, exposure to elevated ambient temperature, hypothalamic damage, malignancies, tissue necrosis, and any other stimulus that could stimulate immune cells to secrete endogenous pyrogens can lead to hyperthermia [22, 23]. Hyperthermia occurs in combination with increased hypothalamic activity with values above the physiological range and occurs when the body's thermoregulatory mechanisms are no longer able to efficiently emit heat (evaporate) [24]. Exogenous environmental stressors, such as high temperature; growth factors and ligands for surface receptors; and many drugs or chemical agents can cause apoptosis. However, cells that have undergone apoptosis show similar morphology, suggesting that these divergent apoptotic stimuli converge to induce a common cell-death pathway. Possible signaling molecules that ultimately lead to apoptosis are interleukin-1-enzyme (ICE)-like1 protease or caspase and other ceramide messengers [25]. If the body temperature of the nucleus does not decrease, a fatal outcome occurs in 30–80% of patients [26]. Heatstroke can cause severe damage to myocardial cells in rats, followed by an increase in apoptotic cells. Heatstroke causes oxidative damage to cellular proteins and DNA [27, 28]. Exposure to heatstroke for 1 hour seriously injures chicken myocardial cells, as evidenced by decreased cell vitality and the onset of apoptosis.

With an increase in body temperature, cardiac output and blood pressure drop drastically and are associated with myocardial oxygen consumption. Hypoxia causes numerous injuries to the heart muscle, from subendocardial hemorrhage, myocardial necrosis, and rupture among fibrin fibers. An increase in internal temperature in rats from 37–42°C also causes tachycardia and increases mean blood flow and vascular resistance by 13% [29]. In the state of heatstroke, large amounts of calcium are released from the sarcoplasmic reticulum of the heart muscle, causing a hypermetabolic state. Continuous increase in calcium allows excessive stimulation of aerobic and anaerobic glycolytic metabolism, leading to respiratory and metabolic acidosis, increased membrane permeability, and the occurrence of hyperkalemia. Rhabdomyolysis leads to an increase in potassium and myoglobin levels in the heart and edema occurs. Disseminated intravascular coagulation occurs as a consequence of thromboplastin release in tissues [30].

1.3 Hematological parameters

Monitoring of hematological parameters enables fast detection of changes in the physiological state because changes in hematological parameters manifest themselves very quickly and precede possible damage. Each species has its own characteristics of individual hematological parameters. It is evident that there are unfavorable endogenous and exogenous factors that can, in certain circumstances, change the original biconcave form of mammalian erythrocytes and thus partially or completely disable its physiological role in gas exchange.

1.4 Erythrocytes: shape and size

Erythrocytes or red blood cells make up the majority of blood cells. Although they are called cells, mature erythrocytes do not have a nucleus, mitochondria, or other organelles. Normal erythrocytes are actually biconcave plates with an average diameter of about 7.8 μm. In the thickest place, their thickness is about 2.5 μm, and in the center 1 μm or less. Their average volume is 90 to 95 μm^3. Their membrane is too large in relation to the cell content, so the deformation will not cause the membrane to stretch, but neither will it burst, which would happen to many other cells. The cytoplasm of erythrocytes contains large amounts of the protein hemoglobin, which is able to temporarily bind gases to itself. It is because of this protein that erythrocytes have the ability to carry oxygen and carbon dioxide.

The total number of erythrocytes in the bloodstream is maintained within relatively narrow limits. The body strives to ensure that the number of erythrocytes is always sufficient to carry oxygen from the lungs to the tissues in appropriate quantities, without impeding blood flow through the blood vessels. Tissue oxygenation is the most important regulator of erythrocyte formation. Any condition in the body that reduces the amount of oxygen in the tissue increases the production of erythrocytes. If a person becomes anemic, due to bleeding or any other reason, the bone marrow immediately begins to produce a large number of erythrocytes. Erythropoietin is a circulating hormone that stimulates the production of erythrocytes, and its production increases in response to hypoxia. Under normal conditions, 90% of erythropoietin is produced in the kidneys and the rest is mostly in the liver. The production of erythropoietin is especially stimulated by adrenaline and noradrenaline, and some prostaglandins. Erythropoietic cells are among the fastest growing and proliferating cells in the human body. Therefore, their maturation and rate of formation are greatly influenced by a person's general nutrition [31].

Erythrocytes, the main carriers of oxygen in the blood, are thought to play a key role in controlling local blood flow to the tissue. According to the hypothesis proposed by Ellsworth et al. (1995), when erythrocytes encounter an area where metabolic requirements are increased, a signaling mechanism associated with oxygen release is triggered, resulting in the release of ATP from erythrocytes into the vascular lumen. ATP acts on endothelial P2y receptors, triggering the release of nitric oxide, prostaglandins, and/or hyperpolarizing factors derived from the endothelium, which in turn act on surrounding smooth muscle cells causing vasodilation [32].

1.5 Poikilocytosis

Poikilocytosis is a term used for abnormally shaped red blood cells (RBCs) in the blood [33]. Poikilocytosis generally refers to an increase in the abnormal shape of red blood cells that make up 10% or more of total red blood cells. Poikilocytes may be flat, elongated, teardrop-shaped, crescent-shaped, may have pointed or thorny protrusions, or may have any other abnormal feature. Examination of the blood smear reveals various forms of erythrocytes. Spherocytes are small round cells that do not have a flat, brightly colored center of regular erythrocytes [34]. The central part of the stomatocyte is incised or elliptical, which differs from the regular round shape of erythrocytes. Dental cells have the shape of a mouth. Podocytes are also known as target cells because they resemble a bull's eye. Sickle cells, also known as drepanocytes, are crescent-shaped and elongated erythrocytes [35]. Elliptocytes, also known as ovalocytes, are oval or cigar-shaped cells with blunt ends. Droplet cells or dacryocytes are abnormal erythrocytes that have one round and one pointed end. Acanthocytes are erythrocytes that have abnormal spike-like protrusions present on the cell membrane. Echinocytes similar to acanthocytes also have protrusions (spicules) on the cell membrane similar to acanthocytes, but the projections in echinocytes are evenly distributed and more frequently present. Schistocytes are fragmented erythrocytes [36–40].

Red blood cells usually carry oxygen and many nutrients to tissues and organs. In poikilocytosis, erythrocytes are irregular in shape and may be unable to carry enough oxygen. Poikilocytosis is caused by other medical conditions, such as anemia; red blood cell membrane defects, such as hereditary spherocytosis; many genetic causes, such as sickle cell disease and thalassemia; eating disorders, such as iron deficiency anemia and megaloblastic anemia; and other causes, such as kidney disease and liver [40].

1.6 Animal model of inducing hyperthermia

The physiological body temperature of rats is from 35.9 to 37.5°C [41]. The body temperature of 40.9°C is the upper limit before the compensating mechanisms are activated [42]. The development of techniques for the induction of hyperthermia in laboratory animals represents a significant contribution to experimental research. According to the available literature, hyperthermia in an animal model can be induced with dry (high temperature) and moist heat (immersion in heated water). Induction of hyperthermia and temperature measurement are important components in heatstroke studies to determine the degree of progression or regression of heatstroke. The electric thermometric method is more suitable and precise for continuous or consecutive measurements in comparison with a classical mercury thermometer. Common temperature measurement sites are the skin, oral cavity, axilla, rectum, and eardrum [43]. The superiority of tympanic measurement over rectal thermometry has not been demonstrated in animal studies.

Until the 21st century, rectal thermometry was the most appropriate technique for measuring temperature in heatstroke studies. At the beginning of the 21st century, the best indicator of the average core temperature of the body is considered to be the temperature of the blood in the pulmonary artery [44]. Due to the poor accessibility of the pulmonary artery, other anatomical locations (esophagus, rectum, and oral cavity) are most often used in the routine measurement of core temperature today [45]. Rats, dogs, monkeys, baboons, cows, rabbits, and sheep were used in experimental studies that allow manipulation of exposure conditions and experimental methodology. Among these species, rats, rabbits, and sheep are the most suitable models because of their resemblance to humans as a reaction to high temperature and given their availability, price, and ease of handling. Such models can be used to simultaneously study different pharmacological and laboratory parameters and functions.

Rats are used for routine experiments, while sheep are reserved only for large experiments in which several parameters and functions of the organism are examined at the same time. Several studies related to heatstroke in rats have been performed as experimental models [46–48]. The models were based on the exposure of rats to high temperatures, dry air, or water, until the core temperature reached a predetermined temperature (40.5°C).

A body temperature value of 40.5°C on exposure for 15 minutes was accepted as a reference for the diagnosis of heatstroke. No direct conditional-consequential relationship between hyperthermia and mortality (less than 10% death) was found in rats exposed to lower temperatures during the experiment [49]. Sharm et al. [50] in their study showed that the animal model for the induction of rat hyperthermia is comparable to the clinical situation. The model has proven useful for studying the effects of diseases associated with exposure to high ambient temperatures on changes in various organs and systems, including the central nervous system. Because hyperthermia is often associated with severe brain dysfunction, additional methods have been described to examine some key parameters of brain injury and the development of brain edema [50]. The research was mostly done for the purpose of proving hypo and hyperthermic therapeutic effects in malignant diseases. Several studies are known to go in the direction of the association between hyperthermia and survival time [47].

The first model of hyperthermia was developed on a dog in 1973 and on a rat in 1976 [51]. Hubbard et al. [47] induced rat hyperthermia by heating the cage at a high temperature and measuring rectal temperature [47]. A study by Weshler et al. [52] investigated the development of thermotolerance in the development of hyperthermia in rats in the aquatic environment. Following the historical sequence, more models of hyperthermia have been developed but most of them cause heatstroke by high-temperature dry air. In the animal model of hyperthermia, a study by Suzuki et al. [1] indicates hyperthermia as a cause of death during bathing and the association between high water temperature and survival time.

In the 19th century, an animal model of piglets was developed to investigate disorders caused by hyperthermia. This experimental study was a pioneer in later studies that demonstrated the role that hyperthermia can play in diseases, such as hemorrhagic shock and encephalopathy syndrome, and, in some cases, sudden infant death syndrome [53–56].

1.7 Cardiovascular response to hyperthermia

When exposed to high temperatures, the circulating flow from the environment is redirected to the skeletal muscles and skin, to give off heat. Acute cardiogenic shock can also occur, leading to intracranial hypertension, cerebral hypoperfusion, cerebral ischemia, and neuronal injury. Prolonged exposure to elevated ambient temperatures can result in convulsions, exhaustion, and heatstroke. Thermoregulatory mechanisms relax, sweating stops, and body temperature rises. A condition accompanied by arrhythmias occurs, and disseminated intravascular coagulation, skeletal muscle, and myocardial necrosis may occur [57]. Rhabdomyolysis, which occurs in such heatstroke conditions, is characterized by rupture and necrosis of striated muscle cells, which can be caused by trauma under conditions of hyperthermia. If rhabdomyolysis is extensive, circulating myoglobin may produce acute renal failure [58]. The mortality rate for such patients exceeds 50%. Death caused by hyperthermia is diagnosed in a hospital or by autopsy mainly using serological and pathohistological methods. Postmortem diagnosis of death caused by hyperthermia and heatstroke presents certain difficulties [59].

Hyperthermia occurs and the result of thermoregulatory mechanisms is felt in many organs, including the heart, which is the first response in the chain. Cardiac dysfunction and degeneration occur secondarily in relation to the massive increase in catecholamine secretion, as well as hyperkalemia, acidosis, and hypoxia [60]. Thanks to the research that has been done, nonspecific abnormalities are noticeable on the electrocardiogram [61], angiograms [62], and pathohistological analyzes of the myocardium [63]. An increase in heart mass due to the hyperthermic effect is also observed [64].

2. Material and methods of research

The study was conducted as a prospective, randomized, controlled, experimental study done on an animal model of causing rat hyperthermia. This study was approved by the Ethical Committee of the Medical Faculty University of Sarajevo under registration number 02–3-4-1253/20, Bosnia and Herzegovina.

2.1 Experimental animals

The experiment used 40 adult albino Wistar rats, both sexes, weighing 250 to 300 g. All animals were kept under the same laboratory conditions, and 7 days before the experiment for acclimatization and adaptation were kept in a vivarium with a 12-hour light regime day-night and at room temperature (20°C ± 2°C). During the experiment, the animals received commercial feed for laboratory animals and running water ad libitum. The care and care of animals, as well as the implementation of all experimental procedures, were carried out in compliance with the International Guidelines for Biomedical Research on Animals-CIOMS (The Council for International Organizations of Medical Sciences) and ICLAS (The International Council for Laboratory Animal Science) [65, 66].

Hyperthermia model was used on 40 adult Wistar rats that were methodologically divided into three experimental groups, depending on water temperature exposure of 37°C (KG, n = 8), 41°C (G41, n = 16), and 44°C (G44, n = 16). Each of the trial groups exposed to 41°C and 44°C water temperature was further classified according to the time of analysis, as the antemortem group (G41-AM; G44-AM) with exposure time of 20 min and the postmortem group (G41- PM; G44-PM) with exposure until time of death.

2.2 Induction of hyperthermia in a rat model

The water bath was filled with water and heated to the target water temperature. The water temperature was continuously monitored on the display with additional measurements with a probe immersed in water and readings on a thermometer. A pre-anesthetized rat with a head above water level, fixed on a wooden board, was immersed in preheated water at the target temperature. Survival times were recorded, which included the time from the immersion of the rats in the water of the set temperature (41°C and 44°C) to the time of death. We defined hyperthermia as an increase in internal temperature by 0.5°C, and heatstroke as an increase in internal temperature above 40.5°C [67] (**Figure 1**).

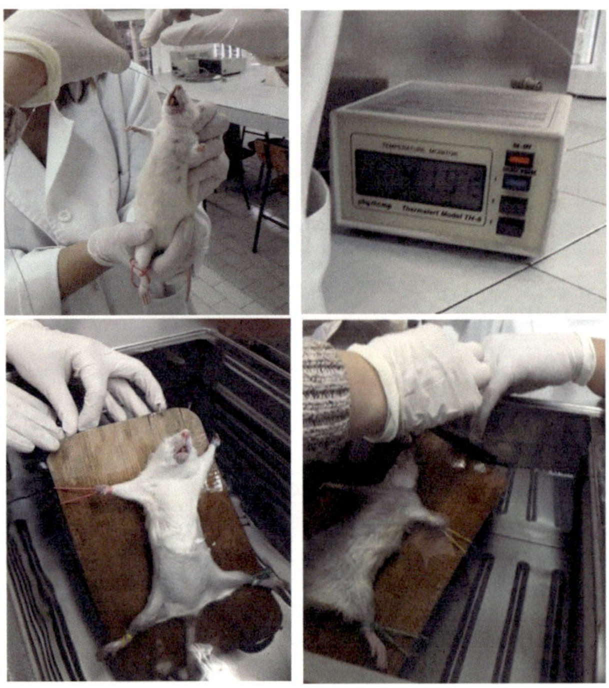

Figure 1.
Experimental procedures in the laboratory of the Faculty of Veterinary Medicine, University of Sarajevo.

2.3 Measurement of heart mass

To measure heart mass, we used a 0.001 mg sensitivity scale (model GT410V, USA) after dissection and before immersion in formalin.

2.4 Microscopic examination and cell counting

Blood samples for analysis were taken from the abdominal aorta. At least two blood smears were made using standard laboratory blood staining techniques (May-Grünwald-Giemsa). Stained blood smears were analyzed by two independent researchers, with counting performed on representative single-layer visual fields where blood cells did not overlap or only touched their edges. Two thousand erythrocytes were analyzed on each stained blood smear using a Motic Type 102 M light microscope and a magnification of 1000 times to examine the presence of poikilocyte red blood cells. The average value of two independent measurements was taken for analysis and the percentages of the number and type of poikilocytes were presented. The most representative microscopic images were stored in electronic form using the software Motic Images Plis 2.0 [68, 69].

3. Results

The body weight of rats in the groups formed according to the length of exposure to elevated temperature ranged from 280.14 g in KG37 to 325.50 g in G44-AM, but there was no statistically significant difference in body weight between groups ($p = 0.081$) (**Table 1**).

The lowest mean heart weight of rats was 0.99 ± 0.11 g in KG37, and the highest value was found in G41 and was 1.15 ± 0.23 g. No statistically significant difference in rat heart weight was found between the three groups, $p > 0.05$ (**Table 2**).

A statistically significant difference in rat heart weight was found in the experimental groups ($p = 0.024$). The lowest value was observed in KG37 and was 0.99 ± 0.11 g, and the highest values were found in rats of the G41-PM group, with a mean value of 1.26 ± 0.26 g (**Table 2**).

Body mass (g)				
Groups	**X**	**±SD**	**95% CI**	
			LL	**UP**
KG37	280.14	43.71	239.71	320.57
G41-AM	315.86	32.29	285.99	345.73
G41-PM	286.75	29.77	261.85	311.65
G44-AM	325.50	47.27	285.98	365.02
G44-PM	281.25	37.90	249.56	312.94

X - mean value; ± SD standard deviation; CI-confidence interval, LL-lower limit; UL-upper limit; KG37-control group of rats exposed to water temperatures of 37°C; G41-AM-antemortem group exposed to water temperature 41°C (exposure length 20 minutes); G41-PM-postmortem group exposed to water temperature 41°C (length of exposure to death); G44-AM-antemortem group of rats exposed to water temperatures of 44°C (exposure length 20 minutes); G44-PM-postmortem group of rats exposed to water temperatures of 44°C (length of exposure to death).

Table 1.
Mean values of body weight of rats in the experimental groups according to the length of exposure to elevated temperature.

The mean values of rat heart weight in the experimental groups differed in the KG37 and G41-PM groups, p = 0.04, and the 41-AM and PM groups, p = 0.08 (**Table 3**).

Table 4 shows the differences in poikilocytotic forms between the antemortem groups (41°C and 44°C) and the control group (37°C).

There is a statistically significant difference between the antemortem group and the control group in ovalocytes, dacryocytes, annulocytes, echinocytes, stomatocytes, spherocytes, reticulocytes, and target cells. Statisticaly significant difference was found between control and antemortem group exposed to 41°C in ovalocytes, spherocytes, reticulocytes, dacryocytes, annulocytes, echinocytes, stomatocytes, and

Group	X(g)	±SD	95% CI		
			LL	UL	P
KG37	0.99	0.11	0.88	1.10	
G41-AM	1.01	0.07	0.94	1.08	
G41-PM	1.26	0.26	1.04	1.48	**0.024**
G44-AM	1.06	0.08	0.99	1.13	
G44-PM	1.15	0.21	0.98	1.33	

X - mean value; ±SD standard deviation; CI-confidence interval, LL-lower limit; UL-upper limit; p-probability; KG37-control group of rats exposed to water temperatures of 37°C; G41-AM-antemortem group exposed to water temperature 41°C (exposure length 20 minutes); G41-PM-postmortem group exposed to water temperature 41°C (length of exposure to death); G44-AM-antemortem group of rats exposed to water temperatures of 44°C (exposure length 20 minutes); G44-PM-postmortem group of rats exposed to water temperatures of 44°C (length of exposure to death).

Table 2.
Mean values of rat heart mass in the experimental groups.

Group	Group	p	95% CI	
			LL	UL
KG37	G41-AM	1.00	−0.29	0.25
	G41-PM	**0.04**	−0.53	−0.00
	G44-AM	0.33	−0.15	0.61
	G44-PM	1.00	−0.34	0.19
	G44-PM	0.73	−0.43	0.10
G41-AM	G41-PM	**0.08**	−0.51	0.01
	G44-AM	1.0	−0.31	0.21
	G44-PM	1.0	−0.40	0.12
G41-PM	G44-AM	0.27	−0.05	0.45
	G44-PM	1.00	−0.15	0.36
G44-AM	G44-PM	1.000	−0.34	0.16

CI-confidence interval; LL-lower limit; UL-upper limit; p-probability; KG37-control group of rats exposed to water temperatures of 37°C; G41-AM-antemortem group exposed to water temperature 41°C (exposure length 20 minutes); G41-PM-postmortem group exposed to water temperature 41°C (length of exposure to death); G44-AM-antemortem group of rats exposed to water temperatures of 44°C (exposure length 20 minutes); G44-PM-postmortem group of rats exposed to water temperatures of 44°C (length of exposure to death)

Table 3.
Multiple comparisons of mean rat heart weight values in the experimental groups.

	A: Temperature 37 C			B: Temperature 41 C			C: Temperature 44 C						
	Med	**Per 25**	**Per 75**	**Med**	**Per 25**	**Per 75**	**Med**	**Per 25**	**Per 75**	**$p^{A v B v C}$**	**$p^{A v B}$**	**$p^{A v C}$**	**$p^{B v C}$**
Ovalocytes	1.0	0.0	2.0	3.50	1.00	6.00	3.00	2.00	3.00	**0.011**	**0.005**	**0.038**	0.155
Dacryocytes	1.0	0.0	2.0	8.50	1.00	12.0	5.00	2.00	9.0	**0.003**	**0.003**	0	0.793
Annulocytes	1.0	0.0	3.0	39.50	31.0	55.0	47.0	25.0	74.0	**0.003**	**0.008**	**0.001**	0.141
Echinocytes	0.0	0.0	1.0	2.50	0.0	38	0.00	0.00	15.0	**0.029**	**0.011**	0.079	0.28
Stomatocytes	1.0	0.0	2.0	10.00	4.0	22.0	17.0	6.00	35.0	**0.001**	**0.003**	0	0.402
Drepanocytes	0	0.0	0.0	0.00	0.0	0.00	0.00	0.00	0.00				
Schistocytes	0.0	0.0	2.0	1.00	1.0	6.00	1.00	1.00	2.00	0.097	0.056	0.079	0.756
Leptocytes	0.0	0.0	0.00	0.00	0.0	0.00	0.00	0.00	0.00				
Acanthocytes	0.0	0.0	0.0	0.00	0.0	1.00	0.00	0.00	0.00	0.687	0.536	0.636	0.867
Spherocytes	1.0	0.0	2.0	1.00	1.0	8.00	2.00	1.00	15.0	**0.023**	**0.019**	**0.007**	0.981
Reticulocytes	1.0	1.0	1.0	1.50	0.0	2.00	1.00	1.00	4.0	**0.027**	**0.019**	**0.02**	0.685
Target cells	1.0	0.0	1.0	24.50	20	34.0	12.0	3.0	24.0	**0.013**	**0.005**	**0.02**	0.375

Variables are represented as median values with an interquartile range. $P^{A v B v C}$ was tested with the Kruskal-Wallis H test, and differences between two groups were tested with the Mann-Whitney U test. P – probability with $p < 0.05$ deemed as significant.

Table 4.
Differences in poikilocytotic forms between antemortem group and control groups.

target cells, while the difference between the control group and antemortem at 44°C exposure is in ovalocytes, annulocytes, spherocytes, reticulocytes and target cell. There was no difference between antemortem at 41°C and 44°C (**Tables 4** and **5**).

When comparing rats' antemortem and postmortem groups exposed to a water temperature of 41°C, there are significant differences in the presence of spherocytes, reticulocytes, and target cells (**Table 6**).

When comparing rats' antemortem and postmortem exposed to a water temperature of 44°C, a significant difference in dacryocytes and spherocytes was observed (**Table 7**).

	Temperature 41°C			**Temperature 44°C**			
	Median	**Per 25**	**Per 75**	**Median**	**Per 25**	**Per 75**	**P**
Ovalocytes	9	4	13	3	1	10	0.094
Dacryocytes	7	5	26	16	8	19	0.481
Annulocytes	50	3	55	100	28	123	0.110
Echinocytes	8	4	59	7	1	13	0.405
Stomatocytes	10	2	51	15	8	26	0.698
Drepanocytes	0	0	0	0	0	0	1.000
Schistocytes	1	1	2	1	1	2	1.000
Leptocytes	0	0	0	0	0	0	1.000
Acanthocytes	0	0	1	0	0	1	0.591
Spherocytes	47	40	84	46	25	54	0.481
Reticulocytes	8	3	11	4	1	10	0.304
Target cells	2	1	4	1	1	2	0.584

Differences in values are tested with Mann-Whitney U test, p - probability with p < 0.05 deemed as significant.

Table 5.
Differences in poikilocytotic forms between postmortem groups at 41°C and 44°C.

	Antemortem			**Postmortem**			
	Temperature 41°C			**Temperature 41°C**			
	Median	**Per 25**	**Per 75**	**Median**	**Per 25**	**Per 75**	**P**
Ovalocytes	3.5	1	6	9	4	13	,051
Dacryocytes	8.5	1	12	7	5	26	,295
Annulocytes	39.5	31	55	50	3	55	,731
Echinocytes	2.5	0	38	8	4	59	,445
Stomatocytes	10	4	22	10	2	51	,731
Drepanocytes	0	0	0	0	0	0	1000
Schistocytes	1	1	6	1	1	2	,945
Leptocytes	0	0	0	0	0	0	1000
Acanthocytes	0	0	1	0	0	1	,836
Spherocytes	1	1	8	47	40	84	**,001***
Reticulocytes	1.5	0	2	8	3	11	**0,041**
Target cells	24.5	20	34	2	1	4	**,001***

**Represents a significant difference between groups.*

Table 6.
Differences in poikilocytotic forms between antemortem and postmortem groups at 41°C.

	Antemortem			Postmortem			
	Temperature 44°C			Temperature 44°C			
	Median	Per 25	Per 75	Median	Per 25	Per 75	P
Ovalocytes	3	2	3	3	1	10	,902
Dacryocytes	5	2	9	16	8	19	**,002***
Annulocytes	47	25	74	100	28	123	,165
Echinocytes	0	0	15	7	1	13	,318
Stomatocytes	17	6	35	15	8	26	1000
Drepanocytes	0	0	0	0	0	0	1000
Schistocytes	1	1	2	1	1	2	,535
Leptocytes	0	0	0	0	0	0	1000
Acanthocytes	0	0	0	0	0	1	,383
Spherocytes	2	1	15	46	25	54	**0,017***
Reticulocytes	1	1	4	4	1	10	,383
Target cells	12	3	24	1	1	2	,053

**Represents a significant difference between groups.*

Table 7.
Differences in poikilocytotic forms between antemortem and postmortem groups at 44°C.

4. Discussion

The aim of the study was to develop and use an animal model of rat hyperthermia and to examine the effect of hyperthermia on erythrocyte shape and heart mass.

The rats included in the study were distributed in groups according to the water temperature to which they were exposed. The bodyweight of rats in groups formed according to the length of exposure to elevated temperature ranged from 280.14 to 325.50 grams (g). Analysis of heart weight by groups did not show a significant difference in the division into three groups according to water temperature, but by division into groups according to water temperature and length of exposure showed that the hearts of postmortem groups had significantly higher mass. The difference between cardiac weight in antemortem and postmortem measurements is due to edema, congestion, and accumulation of blood in the heart cavities as antemortem characteristics and redistribution of blood caused by thoracic dissection during the autopsy, as a postmortem response in cardiac weight [70]. In a study by Michiue et al. [71] in situ cardiac blood volume in cardiac cavities and dilatation index were higher in sudden deaths and lower in cases of bleeding, suffocation, and hyperthermia. In most cases, systolic and/or diastolic function may be reduced in heart failure. Minute volume is also reduced as well as oxygen delivery with vasoconstriction and redistribution of circulating blood. At the same time, due to reduced beating heart volume, renal perfusion is reduced, antidiuretic hormone release is increased, and water and salt retention occur. The result of increased venous pressure is the transudation of fluid into the intercellular space and the appearance of edema. With the gradual development of heart failure, compensatory mechanisms are developed that facilitate the work of the heart and improve the supply of oxygen to the tissues. As a consequence of a long-term compensatory mechanism, the myocardium hypertrophies. This is also a response to the increase in heart weight in groups that have been exposed to hyperthermia for the longest time, and later to heatstroke and experienced death due to exhaustion of compensatory mechanisms. With an increase in body temperature, cardiac output and blood pressure drop drastically and are associated with myocardial oxygen consumption. Hypoxia causes numerous injuries to the heart muscle, from subendocardial hemorrhage, myocardial necrosis, and rupture among fibrin fibers. The effect of hyperthermia on heart weight and erythrocyte shape was studied in rat embryos. An increase in the internal temperature in rats from 37–42°C also causes tachycardia and increases mean blood flow and vascular resistance by 13% [29].

In the state of heatstroke, large amounts of calcium are released from the sarcoplasmic reticulum of the heart muscle, causing a hypermetabolic state. Abnormal forms of red blood cells depending on exposure and length of exposure to higher temperatures have been demonstrated. There is a statistically significant difference between the experimental groups and the control group in ovalocytes, dacryocytes, annulocytes, echinocytes, stomatocytes, spherocytes, reticulocytes, and target cells.

In the antemortem groups (41°C and 44°C) and the control group (37°C), there is a statistically significant difference in almost all poikilocytotic forms, which indicates a direct effect of temperature on erythrocyte shape in 20-minute exposure length in antemortem groups.

Hyperthermia affected changes in the percentage of certain forms of poikilocytes, especially in groups that had longer exposure to high ambient temperatures (aquatic environments). In any case, the thermal process of overheating gives the same effect as a stress reaction that can be caused in different ways and make it a nonspecific reaction.

The lowest temperature at which red blood cells undergo thermal fragmentation is 45°C [72].

In our study, the most pronounced poikilocytotic forms occurred in the postmortem groups at 41°C and 44°C by echinocyte and spherocyte type. In the antemortem group of 41°C, there is a pronounced poikilocytosis for the target cell, which is 100%, while in the antemortem group of 44°C, there is 100% anulocytosis. After statistical analysis between all groups, it is noticed that the number of expressed poikilocytes increased in postmortem groups, that is, with prolonged exposure to high temperatures. In the antemortem groups (41°C and 44°C) and the control group (37°C), there is a statistically significant difference in almost all poikilocytotic forms, which indicates a direct effect of temperature on erythrocyte shape in 20-minute exposure length in antemortem groups.

When comparing antemortem and postmortem rats exposed to a water temperature of 41° C, there are significant differences in some forms of erythrocytes (spherocytes, reticulocytes, and target cells), which suggests that poikilocytosis is more pronounced and associated with the length of exposure to high temperature than temperature between the antemortem and postmortem groups at 41°C. It has been noticed that erythrocytes in organisms that are exposed to heat for a long time are more sensitive and hemolyze very quickly. Their osmotic and mechanical resistance are significantly reduced. The assumption is that the result is damage to the erythrocyte membrane, which becomes permeable, and spherocytes with significantly reduced resistance appear in the blood. Due to erythrocyte damage, hemoglobinemia and hemoglobinuria occur and, consequently, hemolytic anemia. However, unlike erythroptosis, significant hemolysis is activated only at high temperatures with a sharp increase in hemolysis at 41°C and above [73].

When comparing rats exposed to antemortem and postmortem to a water temperature of 44°C, there are significant differences in individual erythrocyte forms (dacryocytes and spherocytes) that agrees with the results of Lucijanović et al. [74]. The higher presence of spherocytes in the blood smear is most commonly associated with anemia and the immune type of hereditary spherocytosis [75]. Mortality can occur at body temperatures of 41°C and above where erythrocytes undergo hemolysis *in vivo*. Metabolic processes within erythrocytes contribute to cell shape change when experiencing suicidal cell death and consequently, nonspecific poikilocytotic forms of erythrocytes occur as a result of hyperosmolarity, oxidative stress, and xenobiotic exposure [76].

Optimal erythrocyte functionality is closely related to ambient temperature. Using digital holography in the microscopic configuration, changes in erythrocyte membrane profile, mean corpuscular hemoglobin (MCH), and cell membrane fluctuations (CMF) of healthy erythrocytes under different temperatures were analyzed. Erythrocytes were exposed to an increase in temperature from 17–41°C for a period of less than 1 hour, after which holograms were recorded. Reconstruction of the obtained holograms showed that there are changes in the 3D profiles of erythrocytes. The amplitude of cell membrane fluctuation was correlated with the curvature curve of erythrocytes, and the changes observed in the indentation of erythrocytes were greater at higher temperatures. Regardless of shape changes, no changes in mean corpuscular hemoglobin concentration were observed with temperature variations [77]. In examining the effect of temperature on syringomycin E pores of lipid bilayer erythrocyte membranes, it was found that different temperatures and pore formation were only slightly affected, while inactivation was strongly influenced by elevated temperature [78]. The movement of erythrocytes through blood vessels at elevated temperature is an interesting and useful task in separating blood cells from the buffer in which they are suspended based on their size or density, and for further analysis. It has been found that increasing the temperature increases the cell-free area near the blood vessel wall due to the inertia of the cell flow after the narrowing of the blood vessel [79]. The movement of erythrocytes through the blood vessel at elevated temperature in this way (increased area without cells near the blood vessel wall), enabled the production of a hybrid microfluidic device that uses hydrodynamic forces to separate human plasma from blood cells. The blood separation device includes an inlet that is reduced by approximately 20 times to a small constrictor canal, which then opens toward a larger outlet canal with a small lateral plasma collection canal. When tested, the device separated plasma from whole blood using a wide range of flow rates, between 50 and 200 microl/min, at higher flow rates injected manually and at temperatures ranging from 23 to 50°C, resulting in an increase in the cell-free layer to 250%. It was also tested continuously using between 5% and 40% of erythrocytes in plasma and whole blood without channel blockage or cell hemolysis. The mean percentage of plasma collected after separation was 3.47% from a 1 ml sample. The change in temperature also affected the number of cells removed from the plasma, which was between 93.5 +/− 0.65% and 97.01 +/− 0.3% at 26.9–37°C, respectively, using the flow rate from 100 microl/min. Due to its ability to work in a wide range of conditions, it is envisaged that this device can be used in *in vitro* "lab on a chip" applications, as well as a hand-held care device (POC) [80].

During cardiopulmonary bypass surgery, perfusion at low temperatures (33–35°C) is recommended to avoid high-temperature cerebral hyperthermia during and after surgery. Also, high body temperatures (40–41°C) affect proteins in both blood plasma and those involved in building red blood cells. The ideal temperature for uncomplicated cardiac surgery is still an unresolved issue. Precisely because of this, the goal of scientific studies was to establish the effect of both low and high temperatures on blood flow and viscosity through blood vessels.

In a study examining the effects of low temperature on blood viscosity, the aim was to determine the effects of temperature, shear rate, hematocrit, and various volume expanders on blood viscosity in conditions that mimic deep hypothermia in cardiac surgery. Dilutions were prepared to 35%, 30%, 22.5%, and 15% hematocrit using plasma, 0.9% NaCl, 5% human albumin, and 6% hydroxyethyl starch. Viscosity was measured in the range of shear rates (4.5–450 s (−1)) and temperature (0–37°C). A parametric expression for predicting blood viscosity based on the studied variables was developed and its agreement with the measured values was examined. Viscosity was higher at low-shear rates and low temperatures, especially at temperatures below 15°C. Reducing hematocrit, especially to less than 22.5%, reduces viscosity. The theoretical model for blood viscosity predicts independent effects of temperature, shear rate, and hemodilution on viscosity over a wide range of physiological conditions, including thermal extremes of deep hypothermia in an experimental setting. Moderate hemodilution to hematocrit of 22% reduced blood viscosity by 30%–50% at a blood temperature of 15°C, indicating the potential to improve microcirculatory perfusion during deep hypothermia [81]. In a study investigating the effects of elevated temperature, it was investigated at which temperature the breakdown of blood plasma proteins occurs after 2 hours of heat exposure. As a result, blood plasma proteins were exposed to heat in the range of 37–50°C for 2 hours. Protein degradation was first established between 43 and 45°C exposure to heat [82]. The importance of the influence of temperature on the cellular elements of blood, its proteins, and thus on its viscosity, has conditioned a large number of scientific researches that have dealt with this problem. Blood viscosity measurements are widely used to monitor patients during and after surgery, which requires the development of a high-precision viscometer that uses a minimum amount of blood. The devices were also used to construct blood viscosity models based on temperature, shear rate, and anticoagulant concentration.

The model has an R-square value of 0.950. Finally, the protein content of the blood can be altered to simulate disease states. Simulated disease states were clearly detected by comparing the estimated viscosity values using the model and the measured values using the device, which demonstrated the applicability of the setting in anomaly detection and disease diagnosis [83]. Taking into account the influence of temperature on erythrocyte shape, blood plasma proteins, and blood viscosity, the optimal temperature for human life activity was determined, assuming that this parameter corresponds to the most intensive oxygen transport in arteries and the most intensive chemical reactions in cells. It was found that oxygen transport mainly depends on blood oxygen saturation and blood plasma viscosity, with both parameters depending on blood temperature and acid-base balance. Additional parameters that affect the volume of erythrocytes and, accordingly, the temperature of the most intensive oxygen transport are taken into account. It is assumed that erythrocytes affect the shear viscosity of the blood in the same way because the impurity particles change the viscosity of the suspension. It has been shown that the optimum temperature is 36.6°C under normal ambient conditions [84].

5. Conclusion

In this study, in antemortem groups, water temperature directly affected morphological forms of erythrocytes, while in postmortem groups, the length of body exposure to high temperature was more important than the direct temperature on the morphological characteristics of red blood cells. Hyperthermia affected the changes in the percentage of certain forms of poikilocytes, especially in the groups that had a longer exposure to high temperatures of the aquatic environment. Heart mass varied with the length of exposure and the duration of debilitating compensatory mechanisms.

Author details

Emina Dervišević[1*], Sabaheta Hasić[2], Lejla Dervišević[3], Zurifa Ajanović[3], Muhamed Katica[4] and Adis Salihbegović[1]

1 Faculty of Medicine, Department of Forensic Medicine, University of Sarajevo, Sarajevo, Bosnia and Herzegovina

2 Faculty of Medicine, Department of Medical Biochemistry, University of Sarajevo, Sarajevo, Bosnia and Herzegovina

3 Faculty of Medicine, Department of Human Anatomy, University of Sarajevo, Sarajevo, Bosnia and Herzegovina

4 Veterinary Faculty, Department of Clinical Sciences of Veterinary Medicine, University of Sarajevo, Sarajevo, Bosnia and Herzegovina

*Address all correspondence to: emina.dervisevic@mf.unsa.ba

References

[1] Suzuki M, Misawa A, Tanaka Y, Nagashima K. Assessment of axillary temperature for the evaluation of normal body temperature of healthy young adults at rest in a thermoneutral environment. Journal of Physiological Anthropology. 2017;**36**(1):18

[2] Yang J, Weng W, Wang F, Song G. Integrating a human thermoregulatory model with a clothing model to predict core and skin temperatures. Applied Ergonomics. 2017;**61**:168-177

[3] Jardine DS. Heat-related mortality. Morbidity and Mortality Weekly Report. 2005;**54**(25):628-630

[4] Sund-Levander M, Forsberg C, Wahren LK. Normal oral, rectal, tympanic and axillary body temperature in adult men and women: A systematic literature review. Scandinavian Journal of Caring Sciences. 2002;**16**(2):122-128

[5] Lepock JR. Cellular effects of hyperthermia: Relevance to the minimum dose for thermal damage. International Journal of Hyperthermia. 2003;**19**(3):252-266

[6] Tansey EA, Johnson CD. Recent advances in thermoregulation. Advances in Physiology Education. 2015;**39**(3):139-148

[7] Natarajan R, Northrop NA, Yamamoto BK. Protracted effects of chronic stress on serotonin dependent thermoregulation. Stress. 2015;**18**(6):668-676

[8] Goda T, Hamada FN. Drosophila temperature preference rhythms: An innovative model to understand body temperature rhythms. International Journal of Molecular Sciences. 2019;**20**(8):1988

[9] Weinert D. Circadian temperature variation and ageing. Ageing Research Reviews. 2010;**9**(1):51-60

[10] Buhr ED, Yoo SH, Takahashi JS. Temperature as a universal resetting cue for mammalian circadian oscillators. Science. 2010;**330**(6002):379-385

[11] Morf J, Schibler U. Body temperature cycles: Gatekeepers of circadian clocks. Cell Cycle. 2013;**12**(4):539-540

[12] Saper CB, Lu J, Chou T, Gooley J. The hypothalamic integrator for circadian rhythms. Trends in Neurosciences. 2005;**28**(3):152-157

[13] Abbott SBG, Saper CB. Median preoptic glutamatergic neurons promote thermoregulatory heat loss and water consumption in mice. The Journal of Physiology. 2017;**595**:6569-6583

[14] Abreu-Vieira G, Xiao C, Gavrilova O, Reitman ML. Integration of body temperature into the analysis of energy expenditure in the mouse. Molecular Metabolism. 2015;**4**(6):461-470

[15] Romanovsky AA. The thermoregulation system and how it works. Handbook of Clinical Neurology. 2018;**156**:3-43

[16] Zhao ZD, Yang WZ, Gao C, Fu X, Zhang W, Zhou Q, et al. A hypothalamic circuit that controls body temperature. Proceedings of the National Academy of Sciences. 2017;**114**(8):2042-2047

[17] Gagnon D, Crandall CG. Sweating as a heat loss thermoeffector. Handbook of Clinical Neurology. 2018;**156**:211-232

[18] Morrison SF, Nakamura K. Central neural pathways for thermoregulation. Frontiers in Bioscience. 2011;**1**(16):74-104

[19] Angilletta MJ, Youngblood JP, Neel LK, VandenBrooks JM. The neuroscience of adaptive thermoregulation. Neuroscience Letters. 2019;**692**:127-136

[20] Rowsey J. Thermoregulation: Cytokines involved in fever and exercise. Annual Review of Nursing Research. 2013;**31**:19-46

[21] Van Breukelen F, Martin SL. Molecular biology of thermoregulation. Journal of Applied Physiology. 2002;**92**(4):1365-1366

[22] Heled Y, Fleischmann C, Epstein Y. Cytokines and their role in hyperthermia and heat stroke. Journal of Basic and Clinical Physiology and Pharmacology. 2013;**24**(2):85-96

[23] Lassche G, Crezee J, Van Herpen CML. Whole-body hyperthermia in combination with systemic therapy in advanced solid malignancies. Critical Reviews in Oncology/Hematology. 2019;**139**:67-74

[24] Yoder E. Disorders due to heat or cold. In: Goldman L, Ausiello D, editors. Cecil Textbook of Medicine. 22nd ed. Philadelphia, Pa: WB Saunders Co; 2004. pp. 626-629

[25] Nixdorf-Miller A, Hunsaker DM, Hunsaker JC. Hypothermia and hyperthermia medicolegal investigation of morbidity and mortality from exposure to environmental temperature extremes. Archives of Pathology & Laboratory Medicine. 2006;**130**(9):1297-1304

[26] Lugo-Amador NM, Rothenhaus T, Moyer P. Heat-related illnesses. Emergency Medicine Clinics of North America. 2004;**22**(2):315-327

[27] Plotnikov EY, Chupyrkina AA, Pevzner IB, Isaev NK, Zorov DB. Myoglobin causes oxidative stress, increase of NO production and dysfunction of kidney's mitochondria. Biochimica et Biophysica Acta. 2009;**1792**(8):796-803

[28] Weber M, Lessig R, Richter C, Ritter AP, Weiß I. Medico-legal assessment of methamphetamine and amphetamine serum concentration–what can we learn from survived intoxikations? International Journal of Legal Medicine. 2017;**131**(5):1253-1260

[29] Nakazawa M, Miyagawa ST, Morishima M, Kajio F, Takao A. Effects of environmental hyperthermia on cardiovascular function in the rat embryo. Pediatric Research. 1999;**30**:6

[30] Walter EJ, Carraretto M. The neurological and cognitive consequences of hyperthermia. Critical Care. 2016;**20**(1):199

[31] Kalsi KK, González-Alonso J. Temperature-dependent release of ATP from human erythrocytes: Mechanism for the control of local tissue perfusion. Experimental Physiology. 2012;**97**(3):419-432

[32] Trangmar SJ, González-Alonso J. Heat, hydration and the human brain, heart and skeletal muscles. Sports Medicine. 2019;**49**(1):69-85

[33] Mangla A, Ehsan M, Agarwal N, Maruvada S. Sickle Cell Anemia. In: StatPearls [Internet]. Treasure Island (FL): StatPearls Publishing; 2021

[34] Zamora EA, Schaefer CA. Hereditary spherocytosis. In: StatPearls [Internet]. Treasure Island (FL): StatPearls Publishing; 2021

[35] Narla J, Mohandas N. Red cell membrane disorders. International Journal of Laboratory Hematology. 2017;**39**(Suppl 1):47-52

[36] Wickramasinghe SN. Diagnosis of megaloblastic anaemias. Blood Reviews. 2006;**20**(6):299-318

[37] Green R, Datta MA. Megaloblastic Anemias: Nutritional and other causes. The Medical Clinics of North America. 2017;**101**(2):297-317

[38] Shah PR, Grewal US, Hamad H. Acanthocytosis. In: StatPearls [Internet]. Treasure Island (FL): StatPearls Publishing; 2021

[39] Martin A, Thompson AA. Thalassemias. Pediatric Clinics of North America. 2013;**60**(6):1383-1391

[40] Manciu S, Matei E, Trandafir B. Hereditary spherocytosis - diagnosis, surgical treatment and outcomes. A Literature Review. Chirurgia (Bucur). 2017;**112**(2):110-116

[41] Delibegovic S, Koluh A, Cickusic E, Katica M, Mustedanagic J, Krupic F. Formation of adhesion after intraperitoneal application of TiMesh: Experimental study on a rodent model. Acta Chirurgica Belgica. 2016;**116**(5):293-300

[42] Režić-Mužinić N, Mastelić A, Benzon B, Mrkotić A, Mudnić I, Grković I, et al. Expression of adhesion molecules on granulocytes and monocytes following myocardial infarction in rats drinking white wine. PLoS One. 2018;**13**(5):196

[43] Tayeb OS, Marzouki ZM. Tympanic thermometry in heat stroke: Is it justifiable? Clinical Physiology and Biochemistry. 1989;**7**(5):255-262

[44] Furlong D, Carroll DL, Finn C, Gay D, Gryglik C, Donahue V. Comparison of temporal to pulmonary artery temperature in febrile patients. Dimensions of Critical Care Nursing. 2015;**34**(1):47-52

[45] Childs C. Body temperature and clinical thermometry. Handbook of Clinical Neurology. 2018;**157**:467-482

[46] Hubbard RW, Bowers WD, Mathew WT. Rat model of acute heat stroke mortality. Journal of Applied Physiology. 1977;**42**(6):809-816

[47] Hubbard RW, Criss RE, Elliott LP. Diagnostic significance of selected serum enzymes in a rat heat stroke model. Journal of Applied Physiology. 1979;**46**(2):334-339

[48] Shido O, Nagasaka T. Thermoregulatory responses to acute body heating in rats acclimated to continuous heat exposure. Journal of Applied Physiology. 1990;**68**(1):59-65

[49] Kielblock AJ, Strydom NB, Burger FJ, Pretorius PJ, Manjoo M. Cardiovascular origins of heat stroke pathophy siology. An anesthetized rat model. Aviation, Space, and Environmental Medicine. 1982;**53**:171-178

[50] Sharm HS. Methods to produce hyperthermia-induced brain dysfunction. Progress in Brain Research. 2007;**162**:173-199

[51] Weshler Z, Kapp DS, Lord PF, Hayes T. Development and decay of systemic Thermotolerance in rats. Cancer Research. 1984;**44**(4):1347-1351

[52] Weshler Z, Kapp DS, Lord PF, Hayes T. Israel Journal of Medical Sciences. 1989;**25**(1):15-19

[53] Zila I, Brozmanova A, Javorka M, Calkovska A, Javorka K. Effects of hypovolemia on hypercapnic

ventilatory response in experimental hyperthermia. Physiology and Pharmacology. 2007;**58**(2):781-790

[54] Kahraman L, Thach BT. Inhibitory effects of hyperthermia on mechanisms involved in autoresuscitation from hypoxic apnea in mice: A model for thermal stress causing SIDS. Journal of Applied Physiology. 2004;**97**(2):669-674

[55] Kiyatkin EA. Brain hyperthermia as physiological and pathological phenomena. Brain Research. Brain Research Reviews. 2005;**50**(1):27-56

[56] White M. Components and mechanisms of thermal hyperpnea. Journal of Applied Physiology. 2006;**101**(2):655-663

[57] Bathini T, Thongprayoon C, Chewcharat A. Acute myocardial infarction among hospitalizations for heat stroke in the United States. Journal of Clinical Medicine. 2020;**9**(5):1357

[58] Danzl DF. Accidental hypothermia. In: Marx JA, Hockenberg RS, Walls RM, editors. Rosen's Emergency Medicine: Concepts and Clinical Practice. 5th ed. St Louis, Mo: The CV Mosby Co; 2002. pp. 1979-1996

[59] Yoder E. Disorders due to heat or cold. In: Goldman L, Ausiello D, editors. Cecil Textbook of Medicine. 22nd ed. Philadelphia, Pa: WB Saunders Co; 2004. pp. 626-629

[60] Gronert GA. Malignant hyperthermia. Anesthesiology. 1980;**53**:395-423

[61] Huckell VF, Staniloff HM, Britt BA, Morch JE. Electrocardiographic abnormalities associated with malignant hyperthermia susceptibility. Journal of Electrocardiology. 1982;**15**:137-142

[62] Huckell VF, Staniloff HM, Britt BA, Waxman MB, Morch JE. Cardiac manifestations of malignant hyperthermia susceptibility. Circulation. 1978;**58**:916-925

[63] Mambo NC. Maligant hyperthermia susceptibility. A light and electron microscopic study of endomyocardial biopsy specimens from nine patients. Human Pathology. 1980;**11**:381-388

[64] Elizondo G, Addis PB, Rempel WE. Stress response and muscle properties in Pietrain (P). Minnesota No. I (M) and PXM pigs. Journal of Animal Science. 1976;**43**:1004-1014

[65] Council for International Organizations and Medical Sciences; World Health Organization. International Ethical Guidelines for Biomedical Research Involving Human Subjects. Geneva, Switzerland: World Health Organization; 2002 preuzeto august 2020

[66] Demers G. "Guidelines for Laboratory Animal Care" — ICLAS President Presentation at the Workshop on Development and Science Based Guideines for Laboratory Animal Care. Washington D.C: National Academies Press; 2003

[67] Kidane AS, Peters R. Heat stroke on the hottest day of the year. Nederlands Tijdschrift voor Geneeskunde. 2020;**1**(6):164

[68] Hori S. Analysis of sudden death during bathing. In: Tokyo Emergency First Aid Association. Report of Committee for Prevention of Accidents during Bathing. Tokyo: Tokyo Emergency First Aid Association; 2001. pp. 39-50

[69] Tochihara Y. Bathing in Japan: A review. Journal of the Human-Environment System. 1999;**3**(1):27-34

[70] Carvalho D, Thomazini J. Morphometric and anatomical evaluation of the heart of Wistar rats. International Journal of Morphology. 2013;**31**(2):724-728

[71] Michiue T, Sogawa N, Ishikawa T, Maeda H. Cardiac dilatation index as an indicator of terminal central congestion evaluated using postmortem CT and forensic autopsy data. Forensic Science International. 2016;**263**:152-157

[72] Choi JW, Pai SH. Changes in hematologic parameters induced by thermal treatment of human blood. Annals of Clinical & Laboratory Science. 2002;**32**(4):393-398

[73] Foller M, Braun M, Qadri SM, Lang E, Mahmud H, Lang F. Temperature sensitivity of suicidal erythrocyte death. European Journal of Clinical Investigation. 2010;**40**(6):534-540

[74] Lucijanić M. Analiza gena i proteina signalnih puteva Wnt i Sonic Hedgehog u primarnoj i sekundarnoj mijelofibrozi (dissertation). Zagreb: Medicinski fakultet Sveučilišta u Zagrebu; 2017. p. 19p

[75] Alloisio N, Maillet P, Carre G, Texier P, Vallier A, Baklouti F, et al. Hereditary spherocytosis with band 3 deficiency. Association with a nonsense mutation of the band 3 gene (allele Lyon), and aggravation by a low-expression allele occurring in trans. Blood. 2011;**88**:1062-1069

[76] Bosman GJ, Willekens FL, Werre JM. Erythrocyte aging: A more than superficial resemblance to apoptosis? Cellular Physiology and Biochemistry. 2005;**16**(3):1-8

[77] Jaferzadeh K, Sim MW, Kim NG, Moon IK. Quantitative analysis of three dimensional morphology and membrane dynamics of red blood cells during temperature elevation. Nature. 2019;**9**:14062

[78] Agner G, Kaulin YA, Schagina LV, Takemoto JY, Blasko K. Effect of temperature on the formation and inactivation of syringomycin E pores in human red blood cells and bimolecular lipid membranes. BBA. 2000;**1466**:79-86

[79] Rodríguez-Villarreal AI, Carmona-Flores M, Colomer-Farrarons J. Effect of temperature and flow rate on the cell-free area in the Microfluidic Channel. Membranes. 2021;**11**:109

[80] Rodríguez-Villarreal AI, Arundell M, Carmona M, Samitier J. High flow rate microfluidic device for blood plasma separation using a range of temperatures. Lab on a Chip. 2010;**10**:211-219

[81] Eckmann DM, Bowers S, Stecker M, Cheung AT. Hematocrit, volume expander, temperature, and shear rate effects on blood viscosity. Anesthesia and Analgesia. 2000;**91**:539-545

[82] Vazquez R, Larson DF. Plasma protein denaturation with graded heat exposure. Perfusion. 2013;**28**:557-559

[83] Khnouf R, Karasneh D, Abdulhay E, Abdelhay A, Sheng W, Fan ZH. Microfluidics-based device for the measurement of blood viscosity and its modeling based on shear rate, temperature, and heparin concentration. Biomedical Microdevices. 2019;**21**:1-10

[84] Guslisty AA, Malomuzh NP, Fisenko AI. Optimal temperature for human life activity. Ukrainian Journal of Physics. 2018;**63**:809-815

Chapter 2

Retinal Disorders in Humans and Experimental ALS Models

Pilar Rojas, Ana I. Ramírez, Rosa de Hoz, Manuel Cadena, Elena Salobrar-García, Inés López-Cuenca, José A. Fernández-Albarral, Lidia Sanchez-Puebla, José Antonio Matamoros, Juan J. Salazar and José M. Ramírez

Abstract

Amyotrophic lateral sclerosis (ALS) is a rapidly progressive neurodegenerative disease that severely impairs the patient's mobility, as it mainly affects the upper and lower motor neurons in the spinal cord. In addition, alterations have also been demonstrated in different parts of the central nervous system (CNS), such as the brain and brainstem. The retina is a projection to the brain and is considered as a "window" to the CNS. Moreover, it is possible to use the retina as a biomarker in several neurodegenerative diseases, even in the absence of major visual impairment. Classically, it was thought that the eyes were not affected in ALS, with respect to extraocular muscles, whereas the remainder of the muscles of the body were distressed. Nevertheless, retinal changes have recently been found in this pathology and could help in diagnosis, follow-up, and even monitoring therapies in this disease.

Keywords: amyotrophic lateral sclerosis, ALS, retina, animal models, SOD1, microglia, protein aggregates, axon pathology, neurodegeneration, neuroinflammation

1. Introduction

Amyotrophic lateral sclerosis (ALS) is the most common progressive motor neuron disease, accounting for 80–90% of all motor neuron diseases cases [1]. Worldwide, the incidence per 100,000 people ranges from 0.3 to 2.5 cases per year [2–5]. Only 10% of the cases are familial [6], ranging from 2 to 15% depending on the population [7], whereas 90% of the cases are sporadic or seemingly sporadic. Overall, both the incidence [8] and the prevalence [9] of ALS vary according to location and race. ALS is more common in men than in women, with a ratio of 1.5:1 [5].

This neurodegenerative disease is rapidly progressive with a typical combination of symptoms of both upper motor neurons (UMNs) and lower motor neurons (LMNs) in different degrees, causing muscle fiber atrophy, which seriously affects the patient's mobility and quality of life [2, 4, 10]. ALS comprises overactive reflexes, as well as muscle weakness and stiffness, and it also involves the swallowing, speech, and respiratory muscles [10–12]. In fact, patients usually die within 2–3 years from diagnosis, frequently due to respiratory failure [5, 13]. The disease usually has a spinal onset, beginning in the extremities and spreading to the rest of the body; however, one in every four patients has a bulbar onset, which has a worse prognosis [4]. ALS is a heterogeneous disease with asymmetrical onset and spreading of UMN and LMN dysfunction, which makes its classification very complex [14]. In addition, no single specific test exists for ALS diagnosis; it is a diagnosis of exclusion based on the initial symptoms, the progression of the disease, and tests to eliminate overlapping conditions.

Although ALS has been considered an exclusively motor disease, over the last few years, several studies have focused on assessing the possible participation of nonmotor areas of the central nervous system (CNS) in this illness. Actually, neuroimaging tests have shown an overall reduction in brain volume, with a loss of focal gray matter and regional white-matter alterations [15–20]. The alteration of these areas leads to cognitive and behavioral changes [16, 18]. During the course of the disease, it has been found that 50% of ALS patients have some degree of cognitive impairment, mainly featuring executive dysfunction and mild memory loss [15, 21].

Classically, it was thought that the eyes were not affected in this disease, with respect to the eye motor muscles, whereas the remaining muscles of the body were affected [22]. However, some studies have found abnormal ocular movements in these patients [23–28]. Nevertheless, this classical concept did not refer to the retina or the optic nerve. Actually, these patients have demonstrated not only abnormal evoked potentials [29–33] but also astrogliosis in nonmotor areas, specifically in the occipital area [34]. Even a significant interocular difference of the P100 in ALS patients was demonstrated in a study of visual evoked potentials [33], similar to the existing asymmetry in the CNS of these patients [14]. Some researchers have also analyzed changes in the visual pathway (a nonmotor neuron area) using optical coherence tomography (OCT) in ALS patients [35–44], finding different changes in the retina and optic nerve, some with contradictory results, stressing the importance of classifying patients by both stage and type of ALS, given the high heterogeneity of the disease.

The retina is considered as an open window to the CNS, and it is possible to use it as a biomarker in multiple neurodegenerative diseases, whether or not there is visual impairment. In recent years, many studies have emphasized the importance of the retina in the diagnosis and monitoring of neurodegenerative diseases, with various pieces of evidence highlighting its value as a biomarker [45–57]. However, what was not so evident was the possible involvement of the retina in neuromuscular diseases, which are chronic progressive neurological diseases, such ALS, that predominantly affect the spinal cord, whereby the neurological involvement is far from the visual pathway.

The purpose of this review is to analyze the retinal changes that have been described in different animal models in this disease, to compare them with each other and to correlate them with the changes described in humans to highlight the possible role of the retina as a biomarker in this disease.

2. Retinal histopathological studies in amyotrophic lateral sclerosis patients and experimental models

ALS is a neurodegenerative disease, which shares some pathophysiological mechanisms common to other diseases of the CNS, such as vascular pathology, glutamate excitotoxicity, fragmentation, aggregation, and functional abnormalities of the mitochondria, impaired retrograde and anterograde axonal structure and transport, increased free-radical and oxidative stress, protein aggregation, and neuroinflammation [12, 58–61]. However, studies in the retina are scarce and have focused only on four such mechanisms, as described below.

2.1 Histopathological studies in ALS demonstrating intraretinal protein inclusions

(**Table 1**, **Figure 1**) Accumulated and altered proteins can interfere with neuronal traffic or can abduct proteins that are essential for proper neuronal functioning causing neurotoxicity [62]. The ubiquitin proteasome system plays an important role in ALS, with reactive ubiquitin inclusions being characteristic of this pathology [5, 63]. Among them, TDP-43 and p62 proteins are specifically indicative of ALS. These inclusions, which are positive for P62 and negative for TDP-43, have been demonstrated in the brain, hippocampus, and cerebellum in ALS patients [64, 65].

There are scarce studies that have focused on the histopathology of retinal tissue in both ALS patients and animal models of mammals with ALS. Actually, the first histopathological analysis in the retina was performed in 2014 on a patient with the C9orf72 mutation. In this study, protein intracytoplasmic p62-positive and pTDP43-negative perinuclear aggregates, typical of ALS/frontotemporal dementia (FTD), were observed in the inner nuclear layer (INL) of the retina [66]. Both the poly-(GA) n dipeptide repeats and ubiquitin in the retina were positively stained for p62, similar to the perinuclear inclusions localized in the brains, specifically in the dentate gyrus, of patients with this mutation [66]. The authors suggested that most of the p62-positive inclusions found were likely placed within the cones of bipolar cells (OFF bipolar cells) and between amacrine and horizontal cells, because they were also stained with GLT-1 and recoverin; in addition, these retinal deposits could be related to the contrast sensitivity impairment manifested by the patient [66]. Moreover, Volpe et al. [67] analyzed two retinas from ALS patients with C9orf72 mutations and demonstrated (i) specific p62 inclusions mostly in the INL (94.9%) and in a smaller proportion in the retinal ganglion cell layer (GCL) (5.1%) in one patient, and (ii) ganglion cell axonal atrophy specifically in the papillomacular bundle in the second patient. On the other hand, abundant positive ubiquilin 2-positive inclusions were also shown in a transgenic mice experimental model with mutant UBQLN2, mostly in the inner plexiform layer (IPL), with a smaller amount in the outer plexiform layer (OPL) and a scarce amount in the GCL. This ubiquilin 2 aggregation in the layers of the retina with more synapses is associated to the ubiquilin 2 accumulation in the dendritic spines of the hippocampus, and it may also be related to the dementia observed in this experimental model. Furthermore, few ubiquilin 2-positive aggregates were detected between the neurosensorial retina and the retinal pigment epithelium, whose appearance was analogous to that of drusen [67]. Similarly, in patients with FTD and progranulin deficiency, lipofuscin deposits were found, sometimes associated with subretinal drusen-like aggregates [68]. Retinal thinning in these patients was detected by OCT before symptoms, suggesting that the eye is affected in progranulin-deficient frontotemporal dementia disease [69].

Eye degeneration was reported in an ALS *Drosophila* model that expressed C9orf72 repeat expansion. The expansion of a noncoding GGGGCC hexanucleotide repeat of the C9orf72 gene on chromosome 9p21 is the most common point mutation in familiar ALS, which generates dipeptide repeat proteins that aggregate in the brain. It is noteworthy that some synthesized compounds revealed a significant biological effect by blocking the neurodegeneration of fly retina at different efficacy levels and upgrading

Mechanism	Author and year	Retinal tissue	Main retinal findings	Other comments
Protein inclusions	Fawzi et al. 2014	One patient with ALS secondary to a C9orf72 mutation	Protein intracytoplasmic p62⁺/TDP43-perinuclear aggregates in the INL	Most of the p62-positive inclusions found were likely placed within OFF bipolar cells and between amacrine and horizontal cells; they may have been responsible for the contrast sensitivity impairment in this patient
	Volpe et al. 2015	UBQLN2P497H TG mice	Ubiquilin2⁺ inclusions mostly in the IPL, with a smaller amount in the OPL and in the GCL	Drusen-like ubiquilin 2-positive aggregates at the level of the sub-RPE space
		Two patients with ALS secondary to a C9orf72 mutation	First patient: Specific p62⁺ inclusions: 94.9% in the INL and 5.1% in the GCL	Second patient: ganglion cell axonal atrophy specifically in the papillomacular bundle
	Azoulay-Ginsburg et al. 2021	ALS fly *Drosophila* model expressing C9orf72 repeat expansion	Eye neurodegeneration	Compounds 9 and 4 of chemical chaperones blocked and upgraded the eye neurodegeneration
Neuroinflammation	Ringer et al. 2017	TG mouse model SOD1G93A	hSOD1⁺ vacuoles in the dendrites of excitatory retinal neurons in the IPL, with hardly any in the GCL and INL	No signs of activation of either the astroglia or the microglia of the retina
	Cho et al. 2019	Mouse model of ALS devoid of Ranbp2	↑ Amoeboid forms and microglial cells surrounding the RGCs	Hypertrophy in RGCs + ↑ metalloproteinases in RGCs + axonopathy in the optic nerve
	Rojas et al. 2021	TG mouse model SOD1G93A (late stage)	Microglial cells activation in retinal tissue	Loss of RGCs
			Cell thickening in the area occupied by each microglial cell	
			↑ Microglial arborization in the area with hyper-ramifications in the inferior sector of the OPL	M1 phenotype or proinflammatory state of microglia: neurotoxic
			Retractions of cells processes + migration and clustering of cells in some areas of the retina	

Mechanism	Author and year	Retinal tissue	Main retinal findings	Other comments
Retinal spheroids and axon pathology	Sharma et al. 2020	Retinal sections of 10 postmortem eyes from ALS patients	PAS⁺ spheroids (> 9.07 μm in diameter) in the RNFL	No significant correlation of retinal spheroids and axon pathology with clinical characteristics of the ALS patients (age at death, gender, disease duration, mode of disease onset, ALSFRS-R, and rate of disease progression)
			P-NF⁺ spheroids (8 to 15 μm in diameter) in the peripheral and pRNFL	
			NP-NF⁺ spheroids (7 to 10 μm in diameter) in the RNFL	
			↑ NP-NF signal in the RNFL and IPL	
Vasculopathy	Abdelhak et al. 2018	34 ALS patients with clinically diagnosed ALS who underwent an OCT	The outer wall thickness of retinal vessels was thicker in ALS patients than in controls	Thinning of the ONL, suggesting a possible impairment of rod and cone function
			There was also no correlation between the vessel measurements and clinical parameters	The whole retinal thickness was negatively correlated with the ALSFRS-R

ALS: amyotrophic lateral sclerosis; FTD: frontotemporal dementia; INL: inner nuclear layer; UBQLN2P497H: dysfunctional ubiquilin 2; TG: transgenic; IPL: inner plexiform layer; OPL: outer plexiform layer; ONL: outer nuclear layer; INL: inner nuclear layer; GCL: ganglion cell layer; sub-RPE: subretinal pigment epithelium; hSOD1: human superoxide dismutase 1; Ranbp2: RAN-binding protein 2; RGCs: retinal ganglion cells; PAS: periodic acid Schiff; P-NF: phosphorylated form of neurofilament; NP-NF: non-phosphorylated form of neurofilament; RNFL: retinal nerve fiber layer; pRNFL: peripapillary retinal nerve fiber layer; OCT: optic coherence tomography; ALSFRS-R: ALS Functional Rating Scale—Revised.

Table 1.
Retinal findings in ALS animal models and patients.

this eye degeneration. The most active chemical chaperones were compound 9, which is a peptide derivative targeted to the endoplasmic reticulum, and compound 4, which is targeted to the lysosome. Consequently, both might be used as a new class of drug candidates to treat ALS and other protein misfolding disorders [70].

2.2 Histopathological studies in ALS and neuroinflammation in retinal tissue

(**Table 1, Figure 1**) Neuroinflammation is a pathophysiological mechanism, which involves the activation of astroglial and microglial cells, and it occurs in many neurodegenerative diseases, such as Parkinson's disease, Alzheimer's disease, ALS, and glaucoma [62]. Microglial cells are the macrophages of the CNS and have the ability to respond to injury by becoming activated; they can proliferate, migrate, and change shape, acquiring an amoeboid appearance in the most active state [62, 71]. On the one hand, in an attempt to protect against damage, microglial cells can secrete proinflammatory molecules, such as interferon γ or interleukin (IL)-1β [62].

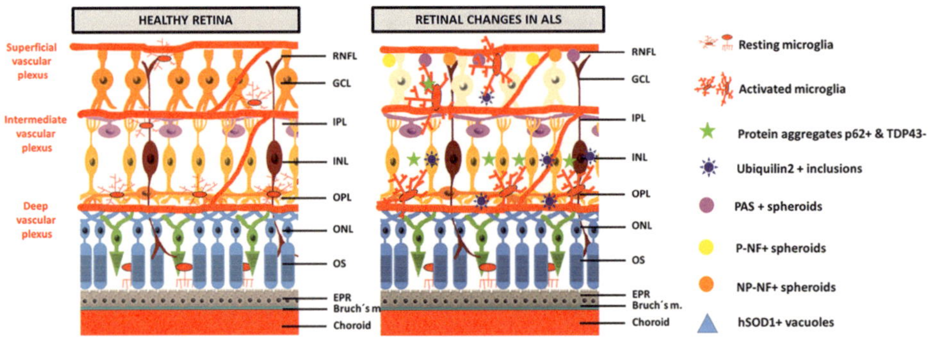

Figure 1.
Summary of retinal changes in amyotrophic lateral sclerosis. (A) Healthy retina. (B) Retinal changes in ALS. Most of retinal changes are mainly detected in the inner layers: (i) ganglion cell loss; (ii) activated microglia in outer plexiform layer (OPL) and inner layer complex (ILC) (constituting an inner plexiform layer and a nerve fiber–ganglion cell layer); (iii) p62-positive and TDP43-negative protein aggregates mostly in the inner nuclear layer with some in the ganglion cell layer (GCL); (iv) ubiquilin 2-positive inclusions mostly in the inner plexiform layer (IPL), with a smaller amount in the outer plexiform layer (OPL) and in the GCL; (v) periodic acid Schiff (PAS)-positive spheroids in the retinal nerve fiber layer (RNFL) and phosphorylated form of neurofilament (P-NF)-positive spheroids in the in the peripheral and peripapillary RNFL; (vi) non-phosphorylated form of neurofilament (NP-NF)-positive spheroids in the RNFL; (vii) hSOD1-positive vacuoles in in the IPL, with hardly any in the GCL and inner nuclear layer (INL).

Nonetheless, uncontrolled activation of the M1 phenotype can lead to a state of chronic inflammation, which can induce neuronal death. On the other hand, microglial cells can also secrete anti-inflammatory molecules, such as IL-10 and the enzyme arginase 1 (Arg1), in order to control inflammation, repair tissue, and improve neuronal survival [62, 71–73]. Consequently, activated microglia can acquire two different activation phenotypes: an M1 or proinflammatory phenotype vs. an M2 or anti-inflammatory phenotype, both of which can be influenced by molecules derived from surrounding cells such as astrocytes [62, 74]. Astrocytes are glial cells of ectodermal origin that perform numerous functions for neuronal survival [75], such as maintenance of the volume and composition of the extracellular space, maintenance of the blood-brain barrier, and regulation of synaptic transmission [76], as well as metabolic maintenance and neuronal survival [77, 78]. When astrocytes are damaged and consequently activated, “astrogliosis” occurs [79]. If this astrogliosis is severe, a glial scar may form [75]. Reactive astrocytes can interact with microglia and neurons and can impair the function of neurons after an injury [80].

Astrocyte activation [81], microglial activation [82], and the appearance of lymphocytes [83] have been found in animal models of ALS (with SOD1 mutations) and in ALS patients. In ALS there are reactive microglia and astrocytes, which can result in motor neuron injury and subsequent death [73, 74, 81]. The SOD1G93A mouse model is one of the most suitable and widely used for preclinical studies in ALS, attributable to the animals having an analogous phenotype to patients. These animals develop limb paralysis due to the loss of motor neurons in the spinal cord, with a reduced lifetime of 150 days [84]. Microglial activation also occurs in ALS, as observed in SOD1-mutated mice and in spinal cord samples from ALS patients, which could exacerbate neuronal damage [73, 74, 81, 85]. In fact, it has been shown that exogenous extracellular mutation of SOD1G93A is not directly toxic to motor neurons, but requires microglial activation for toxicity in primary motor neuron and glia cultures [86]. Furthermore, in SOD1 transgenic mice, activated astrocytes and microglia have been shown to contribute to disease progression but not to disease onset [87–89]. In ALS, microglial activation and proliferation have been observed in areas of significant motor neuron loss, such as the motor cortex, brainstem motor nucleus, corticospinal tract, and ventral horn of the spinal cord [90–94], as well as in areas with mild degeneration [95]. Precisely, in postmortem spinal cord analysis of patients with advanced stages of ALS, reactive astrocytes were found in the dorsal and ventral horn of the spinal cord [96] and in the gray [97] and white matter [34] of the cerebral cortex. Similarly, reactive microglia were found in the motor nucleus of the brainstem, motor cortex, corticospinal tract, and ventral horn of the spinal cord [91]. Reactive microglia were also observed in vivo using the PET imaging technique C-PK11195, finding a close relationship between microglial activation and upper motor neuron damage, but not lower motor neuron injury [98]. Moreover, in the SOD1 model, it was confirmed that overexpression of the SOD1 mutation in glial cells contributes to motor neuron damage, and that the degree of neuronal injury depends on the degree of glial cell pathology [99]. Microglial cells of SOD1-mutated mice suffer different degrees of morphological changes from resting to macrophagic amoeboid forms [91]. Lastly, symptomatic SOD1 transgenic mice also have increased numbers of microglial cells, mainly due to the proliferation of resident microglia [100].

Bearing in mind all of the above, both the microglia and the astrocytes play an important dual role in the progression of the ALS. Nevertheless, most studies about the involvement of microglia in ALS have been conducted in the motor cortex, brainstem motor nucleus, corticospinal tract, and ventral horn of the spinal cord. To our knowledge, there are only three studies that investigated the glial cells of the retina in relation to ALS [101–103].

In the first one, a mouse model of ALS devoid of RAN-binding protein 2 (Ranbp2), microglial activation was confirmed. Ranbp2 is a protein, which plays an important role in nucleocytoplasmic transport and whose regulation is affected in both sporadic and familiar ALS [104]. In this ALS mouse model, there was microglial activation with an increase in the number of microglial cells surrounding retinal ganglion cells (RGCs), as well as a noteworthy increase in amoeboid forms relative to controls. In addition, there was an increase in metalloproteinases in RGCs, and both hypertrophy in RGCs and axonopathy in the optic nerve were found [102].

In the second model, a TG mouse model of ALS SOD1 (SOD1G93A), there was a vacuolization, with hSOD1-positive vacuoles placed in the dendrites of excitatory retinal neurons, which were detected principally in the inner plexiform layer (IPL) and hardly in the GCL and INL; however, no signs of activation of either the astroglia or the microglia of the retina were shown compared with to the wild-type mice [101]. However, the authors did not rule out the possibility that the microglia were undergoing functional changes (in cytokines) related to the inflammatory process. Nevertheless, neuronal changes observed in this SOD1G93A ALS model in the brain at 50 days of age were followed by microglial morphological changes at 60 days [105–107]. Therefore, the authors concluded that, if there is an inflammatory process in the retina, microglia would be in a different, less reactive or even neuroprotective phenotype [101].

Lastly, the third transgenic murine SOD1G93A model of ALS in an advanced stage of the disease (120 days) showed a loss of the number of $Brn3a^+$ RGCs and a microglial activation in retinal tissue [103]. Signs of microglial activation were found in different retinal sectors (superior, inferior, nasal, and temporal) of different retinal layers: outer plexiform layer (OPL) and inner layer complex (ILC) (constituted by an inner plexiform layer and a nerve fiber–ganglion cell layer). In addition, the microglial activation in this SOD1G93A model of ALS showed a cell thickening in the area occupied by each microglial cell, a significant increase in the area of microglial arborization with hyper-ramifications in the inferior sector of the OPL, retractions of cell processes, and migration and clustering of cells in some areas of the retina, but no increase in the number of microglial cells [103]. Moreover, phenotypic analysis of the microglia showed an M1 phenotype or proinflammatory state of microglia, as the cells were intensely labeled with anti-IFNγ and anti-IL-1β but did not stain with the characteristic M2 markers (anti-arginase 1 and anti-IL-10) [103]. The significant decrease in the total number of Brn3a$^+$ RGCs at 120 days of illness would be consistent with the damage observed in the RGCs of the ALS models discussed above [37, 101, 102], as well as with the thinning of the peripapillary retinal nerve fiber layer (pRNFL), observed by OCT, in ALS patients compared with controls [36–44]. Consequently, these data would support that, in ALS, not only are motor neurons affected but also RGC loss occurs, considering this disease as a multisystemic disease [103].

In none of the abovementioned models were changes in the outer segments of the photoreceptors found. This could indicate that neither this layer of the retina nor the outer blood-retinal barrier (BRB) would be compromised in these animals. Because, when the outer BRB is disrupted, as in a glaucoma model of laser-induced ocular hypertension, there are morphological changes and an increase in the number of microglial cells in the photoreceptor outer segment layer [108–112]. Moreover, no changes in the number of microglial cells were found in either the OPL or the ILC [101, 103]; however, the group of Rojas et al. described signs of microglial activation [103]. This difference in results in the same experimental model could be due to the fact that Ringer et al. [101] used retinal sections, while Rojas et al. [103] used retinal whole mounts.

As mentioned above, microglial cells have two distinct phenotypic states that can exert neurotoxic or neuroprotective responses depending on the physiological conditions in which they are found. During ALS progression, activated microglia represent a continuum between the neuroprotective M2 phenotype and the neurotoxic M1 phenotype [113]. In SOD1 ALS animal models, in early stages of the illness, microglia in the lumbar spinal cord expressed markers related to the M2 neuroprotective phenotype (Ym1 and CD206); however, in the late stages of the disease, microglia in the lumbar spinal cord expressed markers related to the M1 neurotoxic phenotype (high levels of NADPH oxidase 2 (NOX2)) [74], suggesting that there is a polarization from a neuroprotective phenotype to a cytotoxic phenotype that induces motor neuron damage. In the retina, there is only one study that analyzed whether microglia are in an M1 or M2 activation phenotype [103]. The results of this study showed that, in 120-day-old SOD1G93A mice, microglia were strongly labeled with antibodies against M1 inflammatory cytokines (IFNγ and IL-1β), but not with those against M2 anti-inflammatory cytokines (arginase-1 and IL-10), suggesting that at an advanced stage of the disease retinal microglial cells are in an M1 activation phenotype or in a pro-inflammatory state that could be neurotoxic to RGCs, as demonstrated by the loss of these neurons. These results are consistent with the findings in spinal cords of the same animal model, where microglia in an advanced stage of the disease showed a neurotoxic M1 phenotype, demonstrating the dual role (neuroprotective/neurodegenerative) of microglial cells during the ALS process [74]. Therapeutic approaches that target microglia polarization and result in the induction of the M2 phenotype are promising strategies to ameliorate local neurodegeneration and clinical outcome of the disease [114].

2.3 Histopathological studies in ALS and retinal spheroids and axon pathology

(**Table 1, Figure 1**) Alterations in axonal transport (retrograde and anterograde) are a hallmark of ALS, being impaired both in ALS patients and in mutant SOD1 mice. In the spinal motor neuron axons, an accumulation of altered mitochondria, neurofilaments, and autophagosomes [12, 58] was demonstrated. On the one hand, mutated dyneins in ALS mice cause this accumulation in the axons of mitochondria and autophagosomes [58]. On the other hand, altered autophagosomes do not eliminate either altered mitochondria or dilated endoplasmic reticules, which accumulate in the axons of motor neurons and cause them to malfunction [12].

There is only one study that focused on this important pathological mechanism in the retina [115]. This study analyzed retinal sections of postmortem eyes from ALS patients with periodic acid Schiff (PAS) and phosphorylated (P-NF) and non-phosphorylated (NP-NF) forms of neurofilament (NF), compared with age-matched controls. Three kinds of spheroids were revealed. First, PAS-positive spheroids with a diameter bigger than 9.07 μm in the retinal nerve fiber layer (RNFL) were observed in most ALS patients (but only in half of controls), most commonly in the pRNFL and the peripheral RNFL, but rarely in the central RNFL in patients with ALS. The density of PAS-positive spheroids was significantly greater in the pRNFL. Second, P-NF-positive spheroids ranging from 8 to 15 μm in diameter were observed in the peripheral and pRNFL only in ALS patients. Additionally, ALS patients showed a stronger P-NF signal intensity in the RNFL in the peripheral, central, and peripapillary regions. Third, NP-NF spheroids ranging from 7 to 10 μm in diameter were observed in the RNFL in some of ALS patients (but not in controls). In addition, in most of the ALS patients, the NP-NF signal was increased in the RNFL and IPL. Nevertheless, there was no significant correlation of these retinal spheroids and axon pathology with the clinical characteristics of the ALS patients (age at death, gender, disease duration, mode of disease onset, revised ALS functional rating scale, and rate of disease progression) [115].

Consequently, patients with ALS show not only hallmark findings in spinal cord motor neurons pointing to disrupted axon transport [116–121] but also retinal spheroids and axon pathology as a shared pathogenesis [115]. Transgenic mice with dysfunctional microtubule-associated motor proteins also display such findings [122–124].

2.4 Retinal vessel pathology and ALS

(**Table 1**, **Figure 1**) Retinal vessels are a reflection of small blood vessels in the brain [125]. Parallel vessel pathology in the retinal and cerebral small blood vessels has been demonstrated in many systemic diseases such as coronary heart disease [126] or stroke [127], as well as in some neurodegenerative diseases such as Alzheimer's disease [128, 129] (even in subjects at high genetic risk of developing Alzheimer's disease [130]) and Parkinson's disease [131].

Some ALS-induced changes have also been described in small blood vessels of the brain, which include a loss of pericytes, endothelial cell degeneration, capillary leakage, downregulation of tight junction proteins, and microhemorrhages in patients with ALS [132, 133]. Moreover, alterations of the structure of small blood vessels of the skin and muscles in ALS patients have been described [134, 135].

There was only one study that analyzed retinal vessel pathology in ALS patients with Spectralis OCT but not with angio-OCT. This study described a thicker outer wall of retinal vessels in ALS patients compared with controls, which may be related to the findings in small blood vessels in skin and muscle biopsies. There were neither significant differences in the vessel diameters between ALS patients with spinal onset and bulbar onset, nor a correlation between the vessel measurements and clinical parameters (disease duration and ALS Functional Rating Scale—Revised (ALSFRS-R)) [136].

3. Conclusions

Much research still remains to be conducted on the retina in both animal models and ALS patients. First, further research should aim to describe the different changes in the retina that occur in all pathogenic mechanisms of the disease. Second, there are several models with different genetic mutations that should also be analyzed. In addition, both the retinal and the choroid changes produced at different times in the evolution of the disease should be studied. It is known that ALS is a heterogeneous disease, with different forms of onset, development, and progression, which may potentially exhibit differences in the retina, as observed in the CNS.

The main findings found in the retina in ALS are summarized in **Figure 1** and **Table 1**.

In conclusion, multiple studies have confirmed that the retina is affected in ALS, mainly in the inner layers, and it could serve as a biomarker in this pathology. These retinal changes can be detected by noninvasive retinal imaging techniques to help in the diagnosis and monitoring of ALS disease. In addition, the retina could be used to evaluate the efficacy of different therapies in ALS in a noninvasive way.

Conflict of interest

"The authors declare no conflict of interest."

Author details

Pilar Rojas[1,2,5†], Ana I. Ramírez[1,3,4†], Rosa de Hoz[1,3,4], Manuel Cadena[2], Elena Salobrar-García[1,3,4], Inés López-Cuenca[1], José A. Fernández-Albarral[1], Lidia Sanchez-Puebla[1], José Antonio Matamoros[1], Juan J. Salazar[1,3,4*] and José M. Ramírez[1,3,5*]

1 Instituto de Investigaciones Oftalmológicas Ramón Castroviejo, Universidad Complutense de Madrid, Madrid, Spain

2 Hospital General Universitario Gregorio Marañón, Instituto Oftálmico de Madrid, Madrid, Spain

3 Instituto de Investigación Sanitaria del Hospital Clínico San Carlos (IdISSC), Madrid, Spain

4 Departamento de Inmunología Oftalmología y ORL, Facultad de Óptica y Optometría, Universidad Complutense de Madrid, Madrid, Spain

5 Departamento de Inmunología Oftalmología y ORL, Facultad de Medicina, Universidad Complutense de Madrid, Madrid, Spain

*Address all correspondence to: jjsalazar@med.ucm.es and ramirezs@med.ucm.es

† These authors contributed equally to this work.

References

[1] Román GC. Neuroepidemiology of amyotrophic lateral sclerosis: Clues to aetiology and pathogenesis. Journal of Neurology, Neurosurgery, and Psychiatry. 1996;**61**(2):131-137

[2] Rowland LP, Shneider NA. Amyotrophic lateral sclerosis. The New England Journal of Medicine. 2001;**344**(22):1688-1700

[3] Sathasivam S. Motor neurone disease: Clinical features, diagnosis, diagnostic pitfalls and prognostic markers. Singapore Medical Journal. 2010;**51**(5):367-372

[4] Kiernan MC, Vucic S, Cheah BC, Turner MR, Eisen A, Hardiman O, et al. Amyotrophic lateral sclerosis. Lancet. 2011;**377**(9769):942-955

[5] Pratt AJ, Getzoff ED, Perry JJP. Amyotrophic lateral sclerosis: Update and new developments. Degenerative Neurological and Neuromuscular Disease. 2012;**2012**(2):1-14

[6] Byrne S, Walsh C, Lynch C, Bede P, Elamin M, Kenna K, et al. Rate of familial amyotrophic lateral sclerosis: A systematic review and meta-analysis. Journal of Neurology, Neurosurgery, and Psychiatry. 2011;**82**(6):623-627

[7] Conwit RA. Preventing familial ALS: A clinical trial may be feasible but is an efficacy trial warranted? Journal of the Neurological Sciences. 2006;**251**:1-2

[8] Haberlandt W. Genetic aspects of amyotrophic lateral sclerosis and progressive bulbar paralysis. Acta Geneticae Medicae et Gemellologiae. 1959;**8**:369-374

[9] Williams DB, Floate DA, Leicester J. Familial motor neuron disease: Differing penetrance in large pedigrees. Journal of the Neurological Sciences. 1988;**86**(2-3):215-230

[10] Yedavalli VS, Patil A, Shah P. Amyotrophic lateral sclerosis and its mimics/variants: A comprehensive review. Journal of Clinical Imaging Science. 2018;**8**:53

[11] Carra S, Crippa V, Rusmini P, Boncoraglio A, Minoia M, Giorgetti E, et al. Alteration of protein folding and degradation in motor neuron diseases: Implications and protective functions of small heat shock proteins. Progress in Neurobiology. 2012;**97**(2):83-100

[12] Zarei S, Carr K, Reiley L, Diaz K, Guerra O, Altamirano PF, et al. A comprehensive review of amyotrophic lateral sclerosis. Surgical Neurology International. 2015;**6**:171

[13] Wijesekera LC, Leigh PN. Amyotrophic lateral sclerosis. Orphanet Journal of Rare Diseases. 2009;**4**(1):3

[14] Zhang Q, Mao C, Jin J, Niu C, Bai L, Dang J, et al. Side of limb-onset predicts laterality of gray matter loss in amyotrophic lateral sclerosis. BioMed Research International. 2014;**2014**:473250

[15] Ringholz GM, Appel SH, Bradshaw M, Cooke NA, Mosnik DM, Schulz PE. Prevalence and patterns of cognitive impairment in sporadic ALS. Neurology. 2005;**65**(4):586-590

[16] Abrahams S, Goldstein LH, Suckling J, Ng V, Simmons A, Chitnis X, et al. Frontotemporal white matter changes in amyotrophic lateral sclerosis. Journal of Neurology. 2005;**252**(3):321-331

[17] Kassubek J, Unrath A, Huppertz HJ, Lulé D, Ethofer T, Sperfeld AD, et al. Global brain atrophy and corticospinal tract alterations in ALS, as investigated by voxel-based morphometry of 3-D MRI. Amyotrophic Lateral Sclerosis and Other Motor Neuron Disorders. 2005;**6**(4):213-220

[18] Mezzapesa D, Ceccarelli A, Dicuonzo F, Carella A, De CMF, Lopez M, et al. Whole-brain and regional brain atrophy in amyotrophic lateral sclerosis. AJNR. American Journal of Neuroradiology. 2007;**28**:255-259

[19] Ellis CM, Suckling J, Amaro E, Bullmore ET, Simmons A, Williams SC, et al. Volumetric analysis reveals corticospinal tract degeneration and extramotor involvement in ALS. Neurology. 2001;**57**(9):1571-1578

[20] Weis J, Katona I, Müller-Newen G, Sommer C, Necula G, Hendrich C, et al. Small-fiber neuropathy in patients with ALS. Neurology. 2011;**76**(23):2024-2029

[21] Meier SL, Charleston AJ, Tippett LJ. Cognitive and behavioural deficits associated with the orbitomedial prefrontal cortex in amyotrophic lateral sclerosis. Brain. 2010;**133**(11):3444-3457

[22] McLoon LK, Harandi VM, Brännström T, Andersen PM, Liu JX. Wnt and extraocular muscle sparing in amyotrophic lateral sclerosis. Investigative Ophthalmology and Visual Science. 2014;**55**(9):5482-5496

[23] Averbuch-Heller L, Helmchen C, Horn AK, Leigh RJ, Büttner-Ennerver JA. Slow vertical saccades in motor neuron disease: Correlation of structure and function. Annals of Neurology. 1998;**44**(4):641-648

[24] Gizzi M, DiRocco A, Sivak M, Cohen B. Ocular motor function in motor neuron disease. Neurology. 1992;**42**(5):1037-1046

[25] Puligheddu M, Congiu P, Aricò D, Rundo F, Borghero G, Marrosu F, et al. Isolated rapid eye movement sleep without atonia in amyotrophic lateral sclerosis. Sleep Medicine. 2016;**26**:16-22

[26] Sharma R, Hicks S, Berna CM, Kennard C, Talbot K, Turner MR. Oculomotor dysfunction in amyotrophic lateral sclerosis: A comprehensive review. Archives of Neurology. 2011;**68**(7):857-861

[27] Shaunak S, Orrell RW, O'Sullivan E, Hawken MB, Lane RJ, Henderson L, et al. Oculomotor function in amyotrophic lateral sclerosis: Evidence for frontal impairment. Annals of Neurology. 1995;**38**(1):38-44

[28] Kang BH, Kim JI, Lim YMKK. Abnormal oculomotor functions in amyotrophic lateral sclerosis. Journal of Clinical Neurology. 2018;**14**(4):464-471

[29] Radtke RA, Erwin A, Erwin CW. Abnormal sensory evoked potentials in amyotrophic lateral sclerosis. Neurology. 1986;**36**(6):796-801

[30] Matheson JK, Harrington HJ, Hallett M. Abnormalities of multimodality evoked potentials in amyotrophic lateral sclerosis. Archives of Neurology. 1986;**43**(4):338-340

[31] Münte T, Tröger M, Nusser I, Wieringa B, Johannes S, Matzke M, et al. Alteration of early components of the visual evoked potential in amyotrophic lateral sclerosis. Journal of Neurology. 1998;**245**(4):206-210

[32] Subramaniam JS, Yiannikas C. Multimodality evoked potentials in motor neuron disease. Archives of Neurology. 1990;**47**(9):989-994

[33] González Díaz N, Escobar Barrios E, Escamilla Chávez C, Escobar RD. Potenciales evocados multimodales en pacientes con esclerosis lateral amiotrófica. Revista Mexicana de Medicina Física y Rehabilitación. 2004;**16**:5-11

[34] Kushner PD, Stephenson DT, Wright S. Reactive astrogliosis is widespread in the subcortical white matter of amyotrophic lateral sclerosis brain. Journal of Neuropathology and Experimental Neurology. 1991;**50**(3):263-277

[35] Roth NM, Saidha S, Zimmermann H, Brandt AU, Oberwahrenbrock T, Maragakis NJ, et al. Optical coherence tomography does not support optic nerve involvement in amyotrophic lateral sclerosis. European Journal of Neurology. 2013;**20**(8):1170-1176

[36] Ringelstein M, Albrecht P, Südmeyer M, Harmel J, Müller AK, Keser N, et al. Subtle retinal pathology in amyotrophic lateral sclerosis. Annals of Clinical Translational Neurology. 2014;**1**(4):290-297

[37] Volpe NJ, Simonett J, Fawzi AAST, Volpe NJ, Simonett J, Fawzi AA, et al. Ophthalmic manifestations of amyotrophic lateral sclerosis (an American ophthalmological society thesis). Transactions of the American Ophthalmological Society. 2015;**113**:1-15

[38] Hübers A, Müller HP, Dreyhaupt J, Böhm K, Lauda F, Tumani H, et al. Retinal involvement in amyotrophic lateral sclerosis: A study with optical coherence tomography and diffusion tensor imaging. Journal of Neural Transmission. 2016;**123**(3):281-287

[39] Simonett JM, Huang R, Siddique N, Farsiu S, Siddique T, Volpe NJ, et al. Macular sub-layer thinning and association with pulmonary function tests in amyotrophic lateral sclerosis. Scientific Reports. 2016;**6**(1):29187

[40] Mukherjee N, McBurney-Lin S, Kuo A, Bedlack R, Tseng H. Retinal thinning in amyotrophic lateral sclerosis patients without ophthalmic disease. Bhattacharya S, editor. PLoS One. 2017;**12**(9):e0185242

[41] Rohani M, Meysamie A, Zamani B, Sowlat MM, Akhoundi FH. Reduced retinal nerve fiber layer (RNFL) thickness in ALS patients: A window to disease progression. Journal of Neurology. 2018;**265**(7):1557-1562

[42] Liu Z, Wang H, Fan D, Wang W. Comparison of optical coherence tomography findings and visual field changes in patients with primary open-angle glaucoma and amyotrophic lateral sclerosis. Journal of Clinical Neuroscience. 2018;**48**:233-237

[43] Rojas P, De HR, Ramirez AI, Ferreras A, Salobrar-Garcia E, Muñoz-Blanco JL, et al. Changes in retinal OCT and their correlations with neurological disability in early ALS patients, a follow-up study. Brain Sciences. 2019;**9**(337):1-18

[44] Zhang Y, Liu X, Fu J, Zhang Y, Yang X, Zhang S, et al. Selective and inverse U-shaped curve alteration of the retinal nerve in amyotrophic lateral sclerosis: A potential Mirror of the disease. Frontiers in Aging Neuroscience | www.frontiersin.org. 2022;**13**(1):783431

[45] Bussel II, Wollstein G, Schuman JS. OCT for glaucoma diagnosis, screening and detection of glaucoma progression. The British Journal of Ophthalmology. 2014;**98**(Suppl. 2):ii15-ii19

[46] Ratchford JN, Quigg ME, Conger BA, Frohman BT, Frohman BE, Balcer LJ,

et al. Optical coherence tomography helps differentiate neuromyelitis optica and MS optic neuropathies. Neurology. 2009;**73**(4):302-308

[47] Dörr J, Wernecke KD, Bock M, Gaede G, Wuerfel JT, Pfueller CF, et al. Association of retinal and macular damage with brain atrophy in multiple sclerosis. Linden R, editor. PLoS One. 2011;**6**(4):e18132

[48] Gordon-Lipkin E, Chodkowski B, Reich DS, Smith SA, Pulicken M, Balcer LJ, et al. Retinal nerve fiber layer is associated with brain atrophy in multiple sclerosis. Neurology. 2007;**69**(16):1603-1609

[49] Siger M, Dziegielewski K, Jasek L, Bieniek M, Nicpan A, Nawrocki J, et al. Optical coherence tomography in multiple sclerosis: Thickness of the retinal nerve fiber layer as a potential measure of axonal loss and brain atrophy. Journal of Neurology. 2008;**255**(10):1555-1560

[50] Stricker S, Oberwahrenbrock T, Zimmermann H, Schroeter J, Endres M, Brandt AU, et al. Temporal retinal nerve fiber loss in patients with spinocerebellar ataxia type 1. Villoslada P, editor. PLoS One. 2011;**6**(7):e23024

[51] Albrecht P, Müller AK, Südmeyer M, Ferrea S, Ringelstein M, Cohn E, et al. Optical coherence tomography in parkinsonian syndromes. Paul F, editor. PLoS One. 2012;**7**(4):e34891

[52] La Morgia C, Barboni P, Rizzo G, Carbonelli M, Savini G, Scaglione C, et al. Loss of temporal retinal nerve fibers in Parkinson disease: A mitochondrial pattern? European Journal of Neurology. 2013;**20**(1):198-201

[53] Schneider E, Zimmermann H, Oberwahrenbrock T, Kaufhold F, Kadas EM, Petzold A, et al. Optical coherence tomography reveals distinct patterns of retinal damage in Neuromyelitis Optica and multiple sclerosis. PLoS One. 2013;**8**(6):e66151

[54] Kesler A, Vakhapova V, Korczyn AD, Naftaliev E, Neudorfer M. Retinal thickness in patients with mild cognitive impairment and Alzheimer's disease. Clinical Neurology and Neurosurgery. 2011;**113**(7):523-526

[55] Gordon-Lipkin E, Calabresi PA. Optical coherence tomography: A quantitative tool to measure neurodegeneration and facilitate testing of novel treatments for tissue protection in multiple sclerosis. Journal of Neuroimmunology. 2017;**304**:93-96

[56] Pfueller CF, Brandt AU, Schubert F, Bock M, Walaszek B, Waiczies H, et al. Metabolic changes in the visual cortex are linked to retinal nerve fiber layer thinning in multiple sclerosis. Kleinschnitz C, editor. PLoS One. 2011;**6**(4):e18019

[57] Bock M, Paul F, Dörr J. Diagnosis and monitoring of multiple sclerosis: The value of optical coherence tomography. Der Nervenarzt. 2013;**84**(4):483-492

[58] Ikenaka K, Katsuno M, Kawai K, Ishigaki S, Tanaka F, Sobue G. Disruption of axonal transport in motor neuron diseases. International Journal of Molecular Sciences. 2012;**13**:1225-1238

[59] Mejzini R, Flynn LL, Pitout IL, Fletcher S, Wilton SD, Akkari PA. ALS genetics, mechanisms, and therapeutics: Where are we now? Frontiers in Neuroscience. 2019;**13**:1-27

[60] Rojas P, Ramírez AI, Fernández-Albarral JA, López-Cuenca I, Salobrar-García E, Cadena M, et al. Amyotrophic lateral sclerosis: A

neurodegenerative motor neuron disease with ocular involvement. Frontiers in Neuroscience. 2020;**14**:566858

[61] Soldatov VO, Kukharsky MS, Belykh AE, Sobolev AM, Deykin AV. Retinal damage in amyotrophic lateral sclerosis: Underlying mechanisms. Eye Brain. 2021;**13**:131-146

[62] Ramirez Sebastian JM. El ojo una ventana al cerebro. An Real Academic Doctors. 2017;**2**(3):357-381

[63] Han-Xiang D, Chen W, Seong-Tshool S, Boycott KM, Gorrie GH, Siddique N, et al. Mutations in UBQLN2 cause dominant X-linked juvenile and adult-onset ALS and ALS/dementia. Nature. 2011;**477**(7363):211-215

[64] Al-Sarraj S, King A, Troakes C, Smith B, Maekawa S, Bodi I, et al. p62 positive, TDP-43 negative, neuronal cytoplasmic and intranuclear inclusions in the cerebellum and hippocampus define the pathology of C9orf72-linked FTLD and MND/ALS. Acta Neuropathologica. 2011;**122**(6):691-702

[65] Williams KL, Topp S, Yang S, Smith B, Fifita JA, Warraich ST, et al. CCNF mutations in amyotrophic lateral sclerosis and frontotemporal dementia. Nature Communications. 2016;**7**(1):11253

[66] Fawzi AA, Simonett JM, Purta P, Moss HE, Lowry JL, Deng HX, et al. Clinicopathologic report of ocular involvement in ALS patients with C9orf72 mutation. Amyotroph Lateral Scler Frontotemporal Degener. 2014;**15**(7-8):569-580

[67] Volpe NJ, Simonett J, Fawzi AA, Siddique T. Opthalmic manifestations of amyotrophic lateral sclerosis (an American ophthalmological society thesis). Transactions of the American Ophthalmological Society. 2015;**113**:1-15

[68] Ward ME, Chen R, Huang HY, Ludwig C, Telpoukhovskaia M, Taubes A, et al. Individuals with progranulin haploinsufficiency exhibit features of neuronal ceroid lipofuscinosis. Science Translational Medicine. 2017;**9**(385):eaah5642

[69] Ward ME, Taubes A, Chen R, Miller BL, Sephton CF, Gelfand JM, et al. Early retinal neurodegeneration and impaired ran-mediated nuclear import of TDP-43 in progranulin-deficient FTLD. The Journal of Experimental Medicine. 2014;**211**(10):1937-1945

[70] Azoulay-Ginsburg S, Di Salvio M, Weitman M, Afri M, Ribeiro S, Ebbinghaus S, et al. Chemical chaperones targeted to the endoplasmic reticulum (ER) and lysosome prevented neurodegeneration in a C9orf72 repeat expansion drosophila amyotrophic lateral sclerosis (ALS) model. Pharmacol Reports. 2021;**73**(2):536-550

[71] Ramirez AI, Rojas B, de Hoz R, et al. Microglia, Inflammation and Glaucoma. In: Glaucoma. SM Group Open Access eBooks. DE, USA: Dover; 2015. p. 1-16

[72] Munder M. Arginase: An emerging key player in the mammalian immune system: REVIEW. British Journal of Pharmacology. 2009;**158**(3):638-651

[73] Philips T, Robberecht W. Neuroinflammation in amyotrophic lateral sclerosis: Role of glial activation in motor neuron disease. Lancet Neurology. 2011;**10**(3):253-263

[74] Liao B, Zhao W, Beers DR, Henkel JS, Appel SH. Transformation from a neuroprotective to a neurotoxic microglial phenotype in a mouse model of ALS. Experimental Neurology. 2012;**237**(1):147-152

[75] De Hoz R, Rojas B, Ramírez AI, Salazar JJ, Gallego BI, Triviño A, et al.

Retinal macroglial responses in health and disease. BioMed Research International. 2016;**2016**:2954721

[76] Perea G, Navarrete M, Araque A. Tripartite synapses: Astrocytes process and control synaptic information. Trends in Neurosciences. 2009;**32**(8):421-431

[77] Bélanger M, Allaman I, Magistretti PJ. Brain energy metabolism: Focus on astrocyte-neuron metabolic cooperation. Cell Metabolism. 2011;**14**(6):724-738

[78] Fernandez-Fernandez S, Almeida A, Bolaños JP. Antioxidant and bioenergetic coupling between neurons and astrocytes. The Biochemical Journal. 2012;**443**(1):3-12

[79] Sofroniew MV. Astrogliosis. Cold Spring Harbor Perspectives in Biology. 2015;7:2

[80] Burda JE, Sofroniew MV. Reactive gliosis and the multicellular response to CNS damage and disease. Neuron. 2014;**81**(2):229-248

[81] Vargas MR, Johnson JA. Astrogliosis in amyotrophic lateral sclerosis: Role and therapeutic potential of astrocytes. Neurotherapeutics. 2010;**7**(4):471-481

[82] Alexianu ME, Kozovska M, Appel SH. Immune reactivity in a mouse model of familial ALS correlates with disease progression. Neurology. 2001;**57**(7):1282-1289

[83] Engelhardt JI, Tajti J, Appel SH. Lymphocytic infiltrates in the spinal cord in amyotrophic lateral sclerosis. Archives of Neurology. 1993;**50**(1):30-36

[84] Gurney ME, Pu H, Chiu AY, Dal Canto MC, Polchow CY, Alexander DD, et al. Motor neuron degeneration in mice that express a human Cu,Zn superoxide dismutase mutation. Science (80-). 1994;**264**(5166):1772-1775

[85] Vinsant S, Mansfield C, Jimenez-Moreno R, Moore VDG, Yoshikawa M, Hampton TG, et al. Characterization of early pathogenesis in the SOD1G93A mouse model of ALS: Part I, background and methods. Brain and Behavior: A Cognitive Neuroscience Perspective. 2013;**3**(4):335-350

[86] Zhao W, Beers DR, Henkel JS, Zhang W, Urushitani M, Julien JP, et al. Extracellular mutant SOD1 induces microglial-mediated motoneuron injury. Glia. 2010;**58**(2):231-243

[87] Philips T, Rothstein JD. Rodent models of amyotrophic lateral sclerosis. Current Protocols in Pharmacology. 2015;**2015**:5.67.1-5.67.21

[88] Yamanaka K, Boillee S, Roberts EA, Garcia ML, McAlonis-Downes M, Mikse OR, et al. Mutant SOD1 in cell types other than motor neurons and oligodendrocytes accelerates onset of disease in ALS mice. Proceedings of the National Academy of Sciences of the United States of America. 2008;**105**(21):7594-7599

[89] Appel SH, Zhao W, Beers DR, Henkel JS. The microglial-motoneuron dialogue in ALS. Acta Myologica. 2011;**30**:4-8

[90] Lampson LA, PD K, Sobel RA. Strong expression of class II major histocompatibility complex (MHC) antigens in the absence of detectable T cell infiltration in amyotrophic lateral sclerosis (ALS) spinal cord. Journal of Neuropathology and Experimental Neurology. 1988;**47**:353

[91] Kawamata T, Akiyama H, Yamada T, Mcgeer PL. Immunologic reactions in amyotrophic lateral sclerosis brain and

spinal cord tissue. The American Journal of Pathology. 1992;**140**(3):691-707

[92] Sargsyan SA, Monk PN, Shaw PJ. Microglia as potential contributors to motor neuron injury in amyotrophic lateral sclerosis. Glia. 2005;**51**(4):241-253

[93] Verine Boillé S, Vande VC, Cleveland DW. ALS: A disease of motor neurons and their nonneuronal neighbors. Neuron. 2006;**52**:39-59

[94] King AE, Dickson TC, Blizzard CA, Woodhouse A, Foster SS, Chung RS, et al. Neuron-glia interactions underlie ALS-like axonal cytoskeletal pathology. Neurobiology of Aging. 2011;**32**(3):459-469

[95] Ince PG, Shaw PJ, Slade JY, Jones C, Hudgson P. Familial amyotrophic lateral sclerosis with a mutation in exon 4 of the Cu/Zn superoxide dismutase gene: Pathological and immunocytochemical changes. Acta Neuropathologica. 1996;**92**(4):395-403

[96] Schiffer D, Cordera S, Cavalla P, Migheli A. Reactive astrogliosis of the spinal cord in amyotrophic lateral sclerosis. Journal of the Neurological Sciences. 1996;**139**(SUPPL):27-33

[97] Nagy D, Kato T, Kushner PD. Reactive astrocytes are widespread in the cortical gray matter of amyotrophic lateral sclerosis. Journal of Neuroscience Research. 1994;**38**(3):336-347

[98] Turner MR, Cagnin A, Turkheimer FE, Miller CCJ, Shaw CE, Brooks DJ, et al. Evidence of widespread cerebral microglial activation in amyotrophic lateral sclerosis: An [11C](R)-PK11195 positron emission tomography study. Neurobiology of Disease. 2004;**15**(3):601-609

[99] Clement AM, Nguyen MD, Roberts EA, Garcia ML, Boillée S, Rule M, et al. Wild-type nonneuronal cells extend survival of SOD1 mutant motor neurons in ALS mice. Science (80-). 2003;**302**(5642):113-117

[100] Solomon JN, Lewis CAB, Ajami B, Corbel SY, Rossi FMV, Krieger C. Origin and distribution of bone marrow-derived cells in the central nervous system in a mouse model of amyotrophic lateral sclerosis. Glia. 2006;**53**(7):744-753

[101] Ringer C, Weihe E, Schütz B. SOD1 G93A mutant mice develop a Neuroinflammation-independent Dendropathy in excitatory neuronal subsets of the olfactory bulb and retina. Journal of Neuropathology and Experimental Neurology. 2017;**76**(9):769-778

[102] Cho K, in, Yoon D, Yu M, Peachey NS, Ferreira PA. Microglial activation in an amyotrophic lateral sclerosis-like model caused by Ranbp2 loss and nucleocytoplasmic transport impairment in retinal ganglion neurons. Cellular and Molecular Life Sciences. 2019;**76**:3407-3432

[103] Rojas P, Ramírez AI, Cadena M, Fernández-Albarral JA, Salobrar-García E, Santos-García I, et al. Retinal ganglion cell loss and microglial activation in a SOD1G93A mouse model of amyotrophic lateral sclerosis. International Journal of Molecular Sciences. 2021;**22**:1663

[104] Ferreira PA. The coming-of-age of nucleocytoplasmic transport in motor neuron disease and neurodegeneration. Cellular and Molecular Life Sciences. 2019;**76**(12):2247-2273

[105] Ringer C, Luisa-Sybille B, MaK S, Eiden LE, Weihe E, Schütz B. PACAP signaling exerts opposing effects on neuroprotection and neuroinflammation during disease progression in

the SOD1(G93A) mouse model of amyotrophic lateral sclerosis. Neurobiology of Disease. 2013;**54**:32-42

[106] Ringer C, Tune S, Mirjam BA, Schwarzbach H, Tsujikawa K, Weihe E, et al. Disruption of calcitonin gene-related peptide signaling accelerates muscle denervation and dampens cytotoxic neuroinflammation in SOD1 mutant mice. Cellular and Molecular Life Sciences. 2017;**74**:339-358

[107] Ringer C, Weihe E, Schütz B. Pre-symptomatic alterations in subcellular βCGRP distribution in motor neurons precede astrogliosis in ALS mice. Neurobiology of Disease. 2009;**35**(2):286-295

[108] de Hoz R, Ramírez AI, González-Martín R, Ajoy D, Rojas B, Salobrar-Garcia E, et al. Bilateral early activation of retinal microglial cells in a mouse model of unilateral laser-induced experimental ocular hypertension. Experimental Eye Research. 2018;**171**:12-29

[109] Rojas B, Gallego BI, Ramírez AI, Salazar JJ, de Hoz R, Valiente-Soriano FJ, et al. Microglia in mouse retina contralateral to experimental glaucoma exhibit multiple signs of activation in all retinal layers. Journal of Neuroinflammation. 2014;**11**(1):1-24

[110] Fernández-Albarral JA, Ramírez AI, De Hoz R, López-Villarín N, Salobrar-García E, López-Cuenca I, et al. Neuroprotective and anti-inflammatory effects of a hydrophilic saffron extract in a model of glaucoma. International Journal of Molecular Sciences. 2019;**20**(17):1-22

[111] Ramírez AI, de Hoz R, Fernández-Albarral JA, Salobrar-Garcia E, Rojas B, Valiente-Soriano FJ, et al. Time course of bilateral microglial activation in a mouse model of laser-induced glaucoma. Scientific Reports. 2020;**10**(1):1-17

[112] Gallego BI, Salazar JJ, de Hoz R, Rojas B, Ramírez AI, Salinas-Navarro M, et al. IOP induces upregulation of GFAP and MHC-II and microglia reactivity in mice retina contralateral to experimental glaucoma. Journal of Neuroinflammation. 2012;**9**(92):1-18

[113] Gordon S, Martinez FO. Alternative activation of macrophages: Mechanism and functions. Immunity. 2010;**32**:593-604

[114] Geloso MC, Corvino V, Marchese E, Serrano A, Michetti F, D'Ambrosi N. The dual role of microglia in ALS: Mechanisms and therapeutic approaches. Frontiers in Aging Neuroscience. 2017;**25**(9):242

[115] Sharma K, Amin MAM, Gupta N, Zinman L, Zhou X, Irving H, et al. Retinal spheroids and axon pathology identified in amyotrophic lateral sclerosis. Investigative Ophthalmology and Visual Science. 2020;**61**(13):8-10

[116] Delisle MB, Carpenter S. Neurofibrillary axonal swellings and amyotrophic lateral sclerosis. Journal of the Neurological Sciences. 1984;**63**(2):241-250

[117] Julien JP. A role for neurofilaments in the pathogenesis of amyotrophic lateral sclerosis. Biochemistry and Cell Biology. 1995;**73**(9-10):593-597

[118] Carpenter S. Proximal axonal enlargement in motor neuron disease. Neurology. 1968;**18**(9):841-851

[119] Munoz DG, Greene C, Perl DP, Selkoe DJ. Accumulation of phosphorylated neurofilaments in anterior horn motoneurons

of amyotrophic lateral sclerosis patients. Journal of Neuropathology and Experimental Neurology. 1988;**47**(1):9-18

[120] Leigh PN, Dodson A, Swash M, Brion JP, Anderton BH. Cytoskeletal abnormalities in motor neuron disease. An immunocytochemical study. Brain. 1989;**112**(Pt 2(2)):521-535

[121] Murayama S, Bouldin TW, Suzuki K. Immunocytochemical and ultrastructural studies of upper motor neurons in amyotrophic lateral sclerosis. Acta Neuropathologica. 1992;**83**(5):518-524

[122] LaMonte BH, Wallace KE, Holloway BA, Shelly SS, Ascaño J, Tokito M, et al. Disruption of dynein/dynactin inhibits axonal transport in motor neurons causing late-onset progressive degeneration. Neuron. 2002;**34**(5):715-727

[123] Laird FM, Farah MH, Ackerley S, Hoke A, Maragakis N, Rothstein JD, et al. Motor neuron disease occurring in a mutant dynactin mouse model is characterized by defects in vesicular trafficking. The Journal of Neuroscience. 2008;**28**(9):1997

[124] Xia CH, Roberts EA, Her LS, Liu X, Williams DS, Cleveland DW, et al. Abnormal neurofilament transport caused by targeted disruption of neuronal kinesin heavy chain KIF5A. The Journal of Cell Biology. 2003;**161**(1):55-66

[125] Patton N, Aslam T, Macgillivray T, Pattie A, Deary IJ, Dhillon B. Retinal vascular image analysis as a potential screening tool for cerebrovascular disease: A rationale based on homology between cerebral and retinal microvasculatures. Journal of Anatomy. 2005;**206**:319-348

[126] Liew G, Wang JJ. Retinal vascular signs: A window to the heart? Revista Española de Cardiología (English Edition). 2011;**64**(6):515-521

[127] Conijn MMA, Kloppenborg RP, Algra A, Mali WPTM, Kappelle LJ, Vincken KL, et al. Cerebral small vessel disease and risk of death, ischemic stroke, and cardiac complications in patients with atherosclerotic disease: The second manifestations of arterial disease-magnetic resonance (SMART-MR) study. Stroke. 2011;**42**(11):3105-3109

[128] Lim JKH, Li Q-X, He Z, Vingrys AJ, Wong VHY, Currier N, et al. The eye as a biomarker for Alzheimer's disease. Frontiers in Neuroscience. 2016;**10**(536):1-14

[129] Salobrar-Garcia E, Méndez-Hernández C, de Hoz R, Ramírez AI, López-Cuenca I, Fernández-Albarral JA, et al. Ocular vascular changes in mild alzheimer's disease patients: Foveal avascular zone, choroidal thickness, and onh hemoglobin analysis. Journal of Personalized Medicine. 2020;**10**(4):1-13

[130] López-Cuenca I, Salobrar-García E, Sánchez-Puebla L, Espejel E, García del Arco L, Rojas P, et al. Retinal vascular study using OCTA in subjects at high genetic risk of developing Alzheimer's disease and cardiovascular risk factors. Journal of Clinical Medicine. 2022;**11**:3248

[131] Kromer R, Buhmann C, Hidding U, Keserü M, Keserü D, Hassenstein A, et al. Evaluation of retinal vessel morphology in patients with Parkinson's disease using optical coherence tomography. PLoS One. 2016;**11**(8):e0161136

[132] Garbuzova-Davis S, Sanberg PR. Blood-CNS barrier impairment in ALS patients versus an animal model. Frontiers in Cellular Neuroscience. 2014;**3**(8):21

[133] Kovács-Öller T, Ivanova E, Szarka G, Tengölics ÁJ, Völgyi B, Sagdullaev BT. Imatinib sets Pericyte mosaic in the retina. International Journal of Molecular Sciences. 2020;**21**:2522

[134] Buckley AF, Bossen EH. Skeletal muscle microvasculature in the diagnosis of neuromuscular disease. Journal of Neuropathology and Experimental Neurology. 2013;**72**(10):906-918

[135] Kolde G, Bachus R, Ludolph AC. Skin involvement in amyotrophic lateral sclerosis. Lancet (London, England). 1996;**347**(9010):1226-1227

[136] Abdelhak A, Hübers A, Böhm K, Ludolph AC, Kassubek J, Pinkhardt EH. In vivo assessment of retinal vessel pathology in amyotrophic lateral sclerosis. Journal of Neurology. 2018;**265**(4):949-953

Chapter 3

Models of Hepatotoxicity for the Study of Chronic Liver Disease

Lourdes Rodríguez-Fragoso, Anahí Rodríguez-López and Janet Sánchez-Quevedo

Abstract

Chronic liver disease affects globally and has a high morbidity and mortality rate. It is histopathologically characterized by the presence of inflammation, and the progressive destruction and regeneration of the hepatic parenchyma, which can lead to the development of fibrosis, cirrhosis, and hepatocellular carcinoma. Most liver diseases tend to become chronic and can be therefore studied in animal models, as it is possible to quickly develop pathological processes in animals with a high degree of reproducibility and obtain predictive data regarding the different hepatopathies. The development of animal models in the field of hepatology has been geared toward the search for new knowledge meant to favor human well-being and proved useful in translational medicine focused on liver disease. Like any other methodological tool, animal models provide valuable. Obviously, a single model cannot reproduce the complexity and spectrum of all liver diseases, which is why a wide variety are currently employed: they include chemically, immune, diet, surgically, and genetically modified damage in animals and involve biological agents or the use of humanized livers in rodents. This chapter surveys some of the main animal models used in the study of chronic liver disease and the disease characteristics they mimic.

Keywords: chronic liver disease, fibrosis, cirrhosis, hepatocellular carcinoma

1. Introduction

Chronic liver disease (CLD) is a major global health problem [1, 2]. Recent studies have shown a global increase in the morbidity and mortality of chronic liver diseases during the past decade [3, 4]. CLD was the cause of an estimated 1.32 million deaths in 2017. Around 1.5 billion people globally are thought to suffer from at least one CLD. The main problem with CLDs is that diagnosis takes place once the disease is already advanced and therapy is no longer as effective [5]. Their treatment also continues to lag behind despite available drug therapies because of three key issues: (1) costly treatments are not accessible to all sectors of the population; (2) the presence of comorbidities such as obesity, hyperlipidemias, or the increase of intravenous drug use and nosocomial spread, just to mention a few, can promote and accelerate the disease, and (3) lack of treatment continuity by either the patient or the health system once the diagnosis has been made. All of these factors play a role in the increase of morbidity and mortality.

Liver cirrhosis is largely due to (1) chronic infection with the hepatitis B virus (HBV) and hepatitis C virus (HCV), (2) alcohol-related liver disease (ALD), and (3) metabolic-associated fatty liver disease (MAFLD) [6–9]. The development of chronic liver disease occurs in different stages: acute hepatic decompensation, multiorgan failure, and compensated and decompensated cirrhosis resulting in higher mortality risks. Decompensated chronic liver disease is associated with the development of hepatocellular carcinoma [10]. Patients with end-stage chronic liver disease or in the hepatocellular carcinoma stage are admitted to hospitals more often, stay in there longer, and are readmitted more often compared with patients suffering from other serious chronic diseases [11]. CLD is a serious illness that entails high medical costs and impacts global public health [12]. It is characterized by extensive production of inflammatory mediators that include cytokines, chemokines, growth factors, bioactive lipid mediators, and immune-mediated tissue damage, all leading to subsequent liver failure [13–17]. The histopathological common denominator, independently of the CLD's origin, is liver inflammation as a mechanism of immune response to hepatocyte injury. Progressive destruction and regeneration of the hepatic parenchyma can lead to the development of fibrosis, cirrhosis, and hepatocellular carcinoma, causing both morbidity and mortality (**Figure 1**) [18–20]. Knowing each of these processes in detail is critical to our understanding of the disease and its therapeutic approaches. Animal models have played an important role in the study of the molecular mechanisms leading to the disease, data collection for early diagnosis, and the evaluation of most of the drugs currently employed in the clinic. Furthermore, they enable the study of new therapeutic alternatives for the prevention and treatment of this group of diseases. This chapter will review the different models employed for the study of the main histopathological and functional alterations that characterize the chronic liver disease. We also include some examples of drugs that have been evaluated using these models.

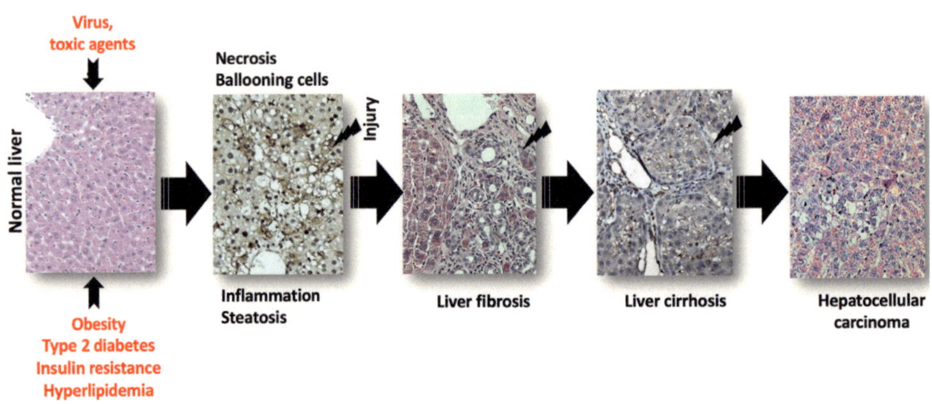

Figure 1.
Progressive necrosis, inflammation, and steatosis of the hepatic parenchyma can lead to the development of fibrosis, cirrhosis, and hepatocellular carcinoma.

2. The importance of animal models in the study of CLD

Throughout history, experimental animals have played a key role in the research of diseases affecting human beings. Rodents are similar to humans in their anatomical, physiological, genetic, molecular, and biochemical conditions, which facilitates studies involving certain diseases. They also incorporate complex factors, such as the environmental and background genetic and molecular changes within a cell under pathological conditions, making them an ideal research tool. From the perspective of scientific research, animal experimentation has contributed considerably to the growth of biomedical science, from the development of prophylactic measures and methods of diagnosis to disease treatments for humans [21, 22]. It can additionally provide information on mechanisms of injury, drug target identification, and characterization of the pharmacological and toxicological profile of innovative drug development.

The best animal model must be easily performed in the laboratory, be reproducible, have no features unrelated to the disease, have minimal limitations, and, most importantly, reproduce both the histopathological and clinical characteristics of the human disease. Poor or inadequate models will result in limited or erroneous information, perhaps even data that cannot be extrapolated to humans. The choice of an experimental model must be precise, as it is the most essential piece in the experimental strategy for the study of liver disease. The most pertinent animal models for CLD research are rodents (rats, mice, and hamsters), but rabbits have been used as well [23]. These animals meet all the basic conditions needed to induce, manipulate, and obtain biological samples for the study of liver disease. Although the choice of the appropriate animal model appears easy, one must take into consideration that it will not completely mimic the human disease because each patient has different and diverse clinical signs and symptoms, comorbidities, genetics, and the complications that might occur from the disease. These conditions cannot be identically mimicked in experimental animals, but it is possible to reproduce the histopathological and functional alterations occurring in the liver tissue. Therefore, the success of CLD studies in animals will depend on the choice of an experimental model that can represent those changes in the liver. Generally, CLD study involves experimentally inducing the disease in the animals, either *via* chemical agents, surgery, genetic modifications, or diet [24]. If the research, however, is focused on mechanisms of injury, specific pathophysiological processes of the disease, molecular targets, pharmacokinetics, or pharmacodynamics, it is important to accurately select species, gender, age, size, number of animals, etc. Said choice will depend on the desired number of samples, organ size, blood volume for the quantification of biochemical parameters and liver enzymes, or obtaining DNA, RNA, etc., for molecular studies. An appropriate experimental animal model enables understanding of the disease, including identification and stage differentiation.

3. Most commonly used models for the study of CLD

CLD is associated with a wide pathological spectrum of alterations, from inactive liver fat storage, associated with an asymptomatic benign clinical course, to progressive cardiovascular, metabolic, and/or liver and kidney diseases with higher cancer risks [25–27]. CLD results from the persistent action of various harmful agents on the liver tissue, exceeding the liver's capacity for defense and repair. The perpetuation of the damage and the liver's response to the damage can produce fat hepatic accumulation without inflammation—an excessive lipid accumulation that induces lipotoxicity accompanied by necrosis and fibrosis development. A constant liver injury might lead more easily to chronicity, as well as a gradual decrease in the hepatocellular mass with subsequent progressive anatomical and functional distortion. From an anatomical point of view, this results in cirrhosis; from a functional point of view, it leads to chronic liver failure. CLD is histologically characterized by the presence of inflammation, steatosis, fibrosis, cirrhosis, and the development of carcinoma (**Table 1**). Therefore, most animal models for the study of liver disease mimic one or more of these histopathological features. We will now address some of the histopathological and functional characteristics of CLD and the animal models that best mimic them.

3.1 Models for the study of inflammation, steatosis, and liver fibrosis

An imbalance between lipid deposition and elimination may lead to hepatic steatosis. There are several cardinal features of hepatic steatosis such as synthesis of triglycerides (TG) and accumulation of free fatty acid (FFA) in the liver. FFA can be processed *via* two different pathways: The first pathway is β-oxidation to generate ATP, and the second is esterification of FFA to produce TG that are either stored within hepatic cells or incorporated into very low-density lipoprotein (VLDL) for release from hepatic cells, thus stimulating an imbalance in fat input/fat output that in turn leads to hepatic steatosis [58].

Histologically, the accumulation of fat in the liver is combined with lobular and periportal inflammation and cell damage (necrosis and ballooning) [59]. Hepatocytes are the main cells involved in the metabolism and mobilization of lipids in the liver. When there is lipid accumulation in hepatocytes, mitochondrial function is overloaded, leading to mitochondrial and peroxisomal dysfunction and increased oxidative stress. Uncontrolled and incomplete lipid oxidation generates toxic lipid products that cause hepatocyte damage and ultimately lead to lipoapoptosis [60, 61]. Apoptosis of hepatocytes can be considered a major cause of liver inflammation, persistent liver damage, and liver regeneration [61, 62]. Chronic inflammation of the liver can induce activation, expression, and signaling of growth factors [63, 64]. As a consequence, the hepatic stellate cells (HSCs) are activated and differentiate from the quiescent phenotype to proliferative and contractile myofibroblasts. Additionally, cells will have the ability to synthesize extracellular matrix [65, 66]. Therefore, a complex network of cytokine-induced pathways arises to coordinate the pro-fibrogenic cell interactions leading to the progression of fibrosis [67–69]. Liver fibrosis is considered a highly complex tissue repair process that appears in the face of sustained hepatocellular damage and that will go through the stages of steatosis, inflammation, regeneration, and liver fibrosis.

Several cells, growth factors, interleukins, receptors, and their signaling pathways participate in the development of CLD and must therefore be analyzed. The study of inflammation, steatosis, and fibrosis can be currently carried out using models that allow for the identification of the typical characteristics of said processes. Models developed for this purpose include diet-induced models, chemical/pharmacologically induced models, and genetic models. Some of the most important features of these models are described below.

3.1.1 Diet-induced models

The diet-induced models include a variety of dietary regimens that range from the administration of substances and fat supplies to caloric intake and additional supplements to facilitate the development of a NASH-like phenotype animal model.

Models	Inductor	Pathology	Advantages
Dietary [28–37]	HFD + CD	Inflammation, steatosis, fibrosis	Resembles human disease and does not require manipulation
	Fructose		
	Cholesterol + fructose		
	Cholesterol + trans fats + fructose		
	MCD	Inflammation, steatosis, fibrosis, cirrhosis, HCC	
	HFD + chemical	Inflammation, steatosis, fibrosis	Fast
Chemical Lee et al., [24, 38–46]	CCl_4	Inflammation, steatosis, fibrosis, cirrhosis, HCC	Fast
	CCl_4 + D-GH + LPS		Advanced fibrosis
	TAA + LPS		Fast
	CCl_4 + DEN		Fast
	DEN		Well tolerated and high HCC incidence
	DEN + TAA		Fast
	DEN + PB	Inflammation, steatosis, fibrosis, HCC	High HCC incidence
	DEN + 2-acetylaminofluorene + PB	Inflammation, steatosis, fibrosis, cirrhosis	Fast
	AS or PS		Lower mortality rates
Genetic [36, 47–54]	*ob*/*ob* mice	steatosis	Well reproducible
	db/*db* mice		
	Zucker *fa*/*fa*		
	SREBP-1 transgenic mice	Inflammation, steatosis, fibrosis	
	PPAR-α Knockout mice	Steatosis	
Surgical [55–57]	BDL	Inflammation, steatosis, fibrosis, cirrhosis	Fast and highly reproducible

HFD, high-fat diet; CD, choline deficiency; MCD, methionine and choline deficiency; CCL_4, AS, albumin serum; PS, porcine serum; carbon tetrachloride; D-GH, D-galactosamine hydrochloride; LPS, lipopolysaccharide; TAA, thioacetamide; DEN, diethylnitrosamine; PB, phenobarbital; BDL, bile duct ligation; HCC, hepatocellular carcinoma.

Table 1.
Models for the study of chronic liver disease.

1. *High-fat animal models.* This group includes the diets characterized by fat intake (up to 70%) with some other combinations such as a diet rich in fat but deficient in choline; a diet rich in fructose intake; a diet rich in cholesterol; a diet rich in cholesterol and fructose; a diet rich in cholesterol, fructose, and trans fats; or a diet rich in fat plus chemicals [28–34, 70]. The advantages are an oral route of

administration, small specimens, and an induction disease time that generally ranges between 12 and 30 weeks. However, the development of some models can be extended for longer periods. This includes a diet deficient in methionine and choline (up to 84 weeks), the high-cholesterol diet (up to 52 weeks), or the chemical diet (up to 52 weeks). The presence of cholesterol in these diets has been reported to increase the severity of the disease [35]. These diets generally lead to the development of steatosis (grade +++), the presence of inflammation (grade ++ or +++), and the development of metabolic syndrome; they are usually employed to address drug discovery or omics data. One advantage of these models is that most can reach the fibrosis stage (grade ++) and some, such as the high-fat diet combined with chemicals, achieve more advanced fibrosis (grade +++) [71, 72]. The development of hepatocellular carcinoma has only been reported with the choline-deficient diet, the high-fat, choline-deficient diet, and the high-fat, high-cholesterol diet [30–32, 70].

2. *The Western/cafeteria diet model.* Other diets try to imitate the bad eating habits that take place among people from big urban centers and with fast food ingestion [73]. These diets are made from a mixture of fat, sugar, and cholesterol. The disadvantage is that they are not standardized and vary greatly across different studies, which makes comparison and reproducibility difficult. There are several combinations that have produced NAFLD using the Western diet method. For example, rats have been fed a 40% fat, 40% sugar, and 2% cholesterol diet for 16 weeks. This diet induced the development of periportal steatosis and inflammation, but there was no development of fibrosis [74]. Another study using hamsters employed a diet containing 40.8% fat, 0.5% cholesterol, and sugar water for 12–16 weeks, leading to the development of microvesicular steatosis, fibrosis, obesity, and insulin resistance. A third study reported a diet based on 40% calories from fat, added sucrose/fructose, and 0.15–2% cholesterol (with and without sugar water) for 24–50 weeks and administered to mice. This study found the presence of steatosis, inflammation, and hepatic fibrosis, as well as obesity and insulin resistance [75]. Although these westernized diets show that the histopathological characteristics of NAFLD can be induced, an analysis of histological patterns, cytokine profile, activation of metabolic pathways, and the degree of damage shows differences in the metabolic profile and hepatic histopathological phenotype [76–78]. Therefore, the extrapolation of these findings to humans is difficult, and these models are not considered adequate for the study of new drugs or for obtaining omics data.

3.1.2 Chemical-induced models

Several studies have reported the use of hepatotoxic agents such as CCL_4, thioacetamide, and diethylnitrosamine to induce NAFLD in rodents. The degree of liver damage varies with the type of agent, the route, and the time of administration. However, said agents have been used for this purpose for over 50 years. CCl_4 is one of the toxic agents that has been widely employed in the research of the liver disease. It can be used by itself or in combination with other agents, either intraperitoneally, orally, by inhalation, or subcutaneously. Its administration ranges from 6 to 12 weeks. The advantage of using this agent is that the histopathological and functional characteristics it produces in experimental animals are already well established. This is one of the models that produces a high degree of steatosis (grade +), as well as a high grade of inflammation and fibrosis (++ or +++), and can even cause portal hypertension and ascites in rodents [38, 39]. In combination with other hepatotoxic, it can lead to hepatocellular carcinoma. Differences in route of administration and dose are associated with variations between research groups. Thioacetamide is a toxic agent that is administered intraperitoneally or in drinking water, achieving liver damage in 10–12 weeks. This agent does not attain a high degree of steatosis, but it produces a high degree of inflammation and fibrosis (grade +++), and even portal hypertension in rodents. However, there have been discrepancies regarding the characteristics of the resulting liver injury. Hepatocellular carcinoma may develop if combined with other agents [40, 41]. Diethylnitrosamine (DEN) is a highly hepatotoxic agent that can be administered orally, intraperitoneally, and in drinking water. It achieves liver damage in 7–18 weeks. The degree of steatosis and fibrosis is very low, but there is a significant inflammatory response [42–44]. Due to its carcinogenic potential, it can lead to hepatocellular carcinoma. These toxic agents can be used as steatosis models for the study of new drugs and to obtain omics data.

3.1.3 Genetic models

Genetically modified animals, by insertion, modification, or deletion of certain DNA sequences, have been widely used for the study of NAFLD and new drug discovery. Genetic models used to study this pathological condition include the following:

1. The *ob*/*ob* mice. These mice do not express leptin and develop hyperphagia, reduced energy expenditure, obesity, hypothermia, and elevated plasma insulin. Obesity in these animals can be observed *via* an increase in adipocyte number and size. Adipose tissue transplants in Lep^{ob} homozygotes guard against obesity, normalize insulin sensitivity, and restore fertility. The main hepatic alterations manifested by these mice include elevations in hepatic mRNA expression for PGC-1α, PPAR-α, an impairment in hepatic mitochondrial function, and a dramatic upregulation in markers of hepatic *de novo* lipogenesis. They show an increase in fatty acid uptake proteins and downregulation of efflux lipid transporters, both of which promote lipid accumulation in the hepatocyte. There is also the recruitment of inflammatory cells, activation of inflammatory signaling pathways, oxidative stress, and lipotoxicity. Animals feeding on a high-fat diet can develop mild perisinusoidal fibrosis in portal areas (week 12) and bridging fibrosis (week 12). The presence of altered hepatic metabolism contributes to the development of NAFLD [47, 48].

2. The *db*/*db* mice are used to model phases 1 to 3 of diabetes type II and obesity. They have polyphagia, are polydipsic and polyuric, and suffer from chronic hyperglycemia, peripheral neuropathy, and myocardial disease. The liver abnormalities observed in these animals include accumulation of fat in the liver (steatosis) and inflammation. Their lipidomic feature indicates the presence of lipid species related to inflammation, energy, and lipid metabolism (FAS, SCD1, LXR β, SREBP-1, and DGAT-1), which leads to lipogenesis and loss of lipid homeostasis. The development of fibrosis in these animals is very low [36, 49]. This model develops neither steatohepatitis nor fibrosis.

3. Zucker *fa*/*fa* rats are the most known and widely used model for the study of obesity. Animals homozygous for the fa allele become noticeably obese by 3 to

5 weeks of age, and by 14 weeks of age, their body composition is over 40 percent lipid. Many metabolic syndrome features, such as hyperphagia, hyperglycemia, hyperinsulinemia, hypercholesterolemia, adipocyte hypertrophy, hyperplasia, and muscle atrophy, can also be observed in this animal model. The presence of an excess in adipocyte mass in these rats, along with insulin resistance, leads to *de novo* lipogenesis and an increased release of free fatty acids up taken by hepatic cells, leading to moderate hepatic steatosis. There is also documented presence of pro-inflammation markers such as TNF-alpha, IL-1beta, and IL-6. This model is more often employed to research inflammation and liver steatosis as associated with obesity [37, 50, 51].

4. SREBP-1 transgenic mice are characterized by the overexpression of the human nuclear sterol regulatory element-binding protein-1c in adipose tissue under the control of the adipocyte-specific aP2 promoter. These genetic alterations lead to an insufficiency of adipose tissue that is evident at birth and is accompanied by severe insulin resistance, leading to symptoms such as hyperinsulinemia and hyperglycemia. These mice exhibit similar 3–4-fold elevations in hepatic nSREBP-1c, which is associated with an increase in mRNAs for several lipogenic enzymes, an increase in the rate of fatty acid synthesis, and triglyceride accumulation in the liver. Liver steatosis is due to endoplasmic reticulum stress induced by SREBP-1 [52, 53, 79]. SREBP-1 transgenic mice are a good model for studying steatosis and steatohepatitis, but not for fibrosis.

5. PPAR-α knockout mice (PPAR$\alpha^{-/-}$) are characterized by high levels of serum triglycerides and extensive hepatic lipid accumulation and plasma fatty acid in plasma. PPAR-α is expressed in the adipose tissue of humans and rodents, stimulating lipolysis in adipocytes. It may also play an important role in regulating whole-body energy metabolism. Contrary to other genetic models, these animals suffer from hypoketonemia, hypothermia, and hypoglycemia but do not present obesity or fibrosis. PPAR-α Knockout mice are the best model for the study of liver steatosis [54, 80, 81].

3.2 Models of cirrhosis and hepatocellular carcinoma

The main complication of CLD is cirrhosis [82]. Liver cirrhosis is a chronic, diffuse, and irreversible liver disease characterized by the existence of fibrosis, portal hypertension, and regenerative nodules. As a consequence, there are fewer liver cells and the liver stops carrying out its usual functions, including the synthesis of proteins (especially those that act in blood coagulation), the production of bile, the neutralization and elimination of foreign substances from the body, and the production of defenses against infection [83]. Although their clinical, biological, and laboratory manifestations can often suggest what the diagnosis is, this can only be confirmed *via* morphological study (biopsy). The prognosis is poor, and patients die from gastrointestinal bleeding, hepatocellular failure, neoplastic degeneration, or metastasis [84].

The development of hepatocellular carcinoma is common in the evolution of patients with liver cirrhosis [85]. Once cirrhosis is diagnosed, the chance of developing hepatocellular carcinoma is of 20% during the following 5 years. Since this type of carcinoma is frequently derived from cirrhosis, its clinical manifestations are often codependent. Prognosis depends on the evolution of cirrhosis at the time the cancer is diagnosed. If hepatic functional reserve is good and hepatocellular carcinoma is asymptomatic, the patient may survive for several years. If the cirrhosis is very advanced and the carcinoma is very developed, the patient will die in a matter of weeks [86].

Chemically induced animal models are most often used for the study of cirrhosis and hepatocellular carcinoma, and some have already been mentioned above. However, to achieve the development of cirrhosis, portal hypertension, or liver cancer, it is necessary to extend the exposure time to the toxic agent, and there are other models specifically focused on the development of liver cirrhosis or hepatocellular carcinoma (**Figure 2**).

3.2.1 Chemical-induced models

CCl_4 in combination with D-galactosamine hydrochloride (GaIN) with or without lipopolysaccharides (LPS) is one of the more often employed models for developing liver cirrhosis. LPS is added to activate Kupffer cells and stimulate TNF-α, as well as an immune response *via* NF-κB pathway activation. D-galactosamine is used to potentiate this response by depleting the uridine nucleotides and interfering in protein synthesis, leading to acute lesions as a precipitating event [87]. Liver cirrhosis is developed in 10 weeks. In this model, we see an increase in aspartate amino transferase (AST) and alanine amino transferase (ALT), as well as the presence of necrosis, and excessive fibrosis and regenerative nodules. Thioacetamide combined with LPS has been used to induce decompensated cirrhosis. After 10 weeks of its administration in the drinking water, increases in liver enzymes, portal hypertension, fibrosis, and cirrhosis can be observed.

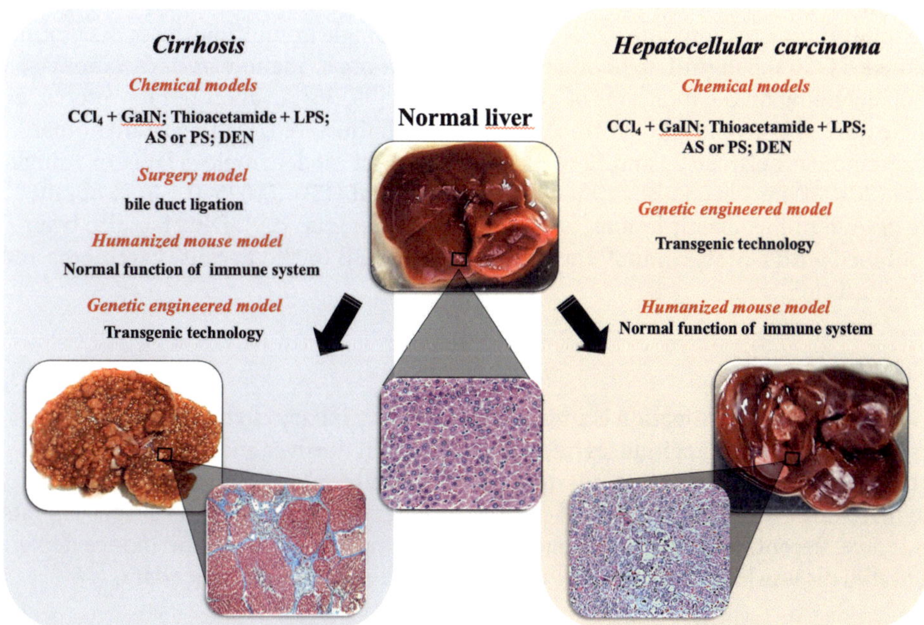

Figure 2.
Models of cirrhosis and hepatocellular carcinoma. Examples of animal models to induce cirrhosis and hepatocellular carcinoma: chemicals, surgery, genetic engineering, and humanized mice. CCl_4: carbon tetrachloride; GaIN: D-galactosamine hydrochloride; LPS: lipopolysaccharides; AS: albumin serum; PS; porcine serum; DEN: diethylnitrosamine.

Albumin serum (AS) and porcine serum (PS) administrations are two other potential models for inducing immune cirrhosis. Albumin becomes hepatotoxic when there is an imbalance of it in the liver [88]. Albumin or PS may induce cirrhosis when interacting with LPS or when undergoing irreversible alkalization *via* drug metabolization. The administration of albumin or PS twice a week for 6 weeks leads to CLD decompensation and subsequent histological and functional liver changes. There is also an increase in several inflammatory markers, such as IL-6, IL-18, and HMGB-1 [89]. The PS model may be more adequate for the induction of immune cirrhosis. It induces a response that is closer to human liver disease, is easier to manipulate, and results in lower mortality rates for animals when compared with the other mentioned models.

DEN is the most important and widely used toxic agent for the development of chemically induced HCC in rodents. It is a carcinogen, and DEN bioactivation occurs in the liver *via* cytochrome P450 (CYP 2E1) [90]. DEN is metabolized *via* alpha-hydroxylation and dealkylation reactions, producing an unstable ethyldiazonium hydroxide molecule that can generate highly reactive carbon, oxygen (ROS), and nitrogen (RNS) ion species. These reactive molecules bind to DNA and proteins and can contribute to genomic instability, DNA damage, mutation, and tumor initiation [91]. DEN "initiates" the hepatocarcinogenesis process and produces a stable and heritable mutational change in hepatocytes, inducing genomic alterations in oncogenes and tumor suppressor genes. HCC can clonally expand from this single DEN-"initiated" hepatocyte and result in HCC.

There are different protocols where DEN is used to induce HCC in rodents. For example, it can be administered alone and in single intraperitoneal doses ranging from 1 to 5 mg, resulting in adenomas (0–20%) in 24 weeks or carcinoma in 36 to 52 weeks [92–94]. When administered in multiple doses, it is used in doses of 25 to 50 mg for 4–8 weeks, resulting in preneoplastic lesions, adenoma, or carcinoma depending on the total administration time. DEN may be used in single or multiple doses in combination with CCl_4 0.5 mg/mL to obtain preneoplastic lesions, adenomas, or carcinomas, also depending on the total time of administration [95, 96]. In another rat protocol, a single dose of DEN plus 0.03% thioacetamide is administered, leading to adenomas or carcinomas between 24 and 52 weeks [97, 98]. A rat model employs DEN in a single dose (80–200 mg) in combination with phenobarbital (PB) (0.025–0.1%) to obtain the desired preneoplastic lesions, adenomas, or carcinomas [99]. DEN has also been combined with 2-acetylaminofluorene (0.02%) and PB (67%) to cause carcinoma and metastasis [45].

3.2.2 Surgery model

Common bile duct ligation is a model of secondary biliary cirrhosis. The surgical resection of the bile duct induces bile accumulation in the liver and thus leads to damage, inflammation, fibrosis, portal inflammation, and cirrhosis after 2 weeks [46, 55]. An increase in AST, ALT, and total bilirubin levels can be observed after surgery in rats and mice. Recent reports suggest that the use of a single dose of LPS can induce decompensated disease [56]. This model is used for drug discovery and omics data.

3.2.3 Genetically engineered models

The above-mentioned models have been in use for more than 30 years and allow for a deeper understanding of the pathogenic mechanisms involved in chronic liver disease and malignant transformation. The better known genetically engineered models include HBV-transgenic, HCV-transgenic, *c-myc*-transgenic, *c-myc*-/TGF-α transgenic, E2F-1 transgenic, *c-myc*-/E2F-1 transgenic, *Apc* knockout mice, β-catenin/H-ras mutant, and cMyc+shp53 mice. Transgenic technology was initiated by inserting exogenous viral DNA into mice to induce the expression of different components of the viral particle [57]. Afterward, several important protein-coding genes and transcriptional enhancers associated with cancer were micro-injected into single-cell embryos of specific mice strains. Most transgenic mice show micro- and macro-fat vacuoles (at 6 and 11 months of age). Although inflammation is not commonly observed between 6 and 15 months of age, most mice develop preneoplastic hepatic lesions and adenomas at 6 and 11 months [100]. Those changes are accompanied by alterations in glycolysis and lipogenesis, which play a key role in the early (preneoplastic) stages of hepatocarcinogenesis. A high incidence of adenomas and carcinomas appears between 40 and 136 weeks. The advantage of these models is that they are highly reproducible and resemble human disease.

3.2.4 Humanized mouse model

Humanized mouse models are widely used to mimic the human immune system in mice [101]. This mouse model is based on transplanted human cells and tissues that have been uniquely engineered to produce combinations of human cytokines in immunocompromised mice and avoid rejection of implanted cells. This kind of model results in a more physiologically relevant model system for evaluating new cancer therapies, immuno-oncology, and effective treatments targeting the tumor microenvironment. Proteomics studies of humanized models have shown that there is an increase in proteins related to apoptosis at 12 months, the defense of fatty acid metabolism against oxidative stress [102]. Other studies have shown that, in combination with DEN, there can be an increase in the size of neoplastic nodules [103]. The mouse is the most widely used animal model in biomedical research because it is versatile, inexpensive, and genetically very similar to humans. However, success depends on animal age, sex, and strain.

4. Regulatory issues regarding the use of animal models in CLD research

Biotechnological advances in medicine and pharmaceutical sciences during recent decades have provided us with tools for better diagnosis and treatment of CLD. This has gone hand in hand with the exponential rise in the use of animal models for research. Animal models in preclinical trials have largely served as the scientific basis for the data that has enabled a better understanding of the pathophysiology of human disease. However, researchers around the world are currently expressing concern about the use of animals for scientific experimentation [104].

To make use of animal models in the field of hepatology, as well as in other medical areas, we must essentially consider various aspects regarding the rational use and management of animals for their use in research protocols. Whenever animals are used as research models, we must keep in mind that the main purpose of the study is to obtain feasible, reproducible, and reliable results inasmuch CLD comprises an important health problem that requires prompt study and attention. One way to achieve this is to reduce the stress to which animals are subjected throughout the study. Aforesaid, the induction of the different stages of CLD requires handling the animals for prolonged periods of time, which can affect and compromise animal welfare. On the other hand, we already know that stress influences affective behavior and stress hormone release may alter the pathophysiology of the CLD [105–108]. For this reason, the scientific community has been made aware of the importance of ensuring the socio-environmental welfare of experimental animals. In Europe, for example, there are regulations regarding the use of experimental animals and a series of standards have been established regarding protection criteria and ethical issues. The scientific community has always been encouraged to implement them insofar as this is possible [109].

Discussions regarding the use of animal models are not recent and have increased over the years, involving the scientific community across different countries [110–112]. Today, there are standards such as Animals in Research: Reporting In Vivo Experiments (ARRIVE), which, since 2010, has become a useful guideline in biomedical science and related areas and is meant to improve the use and management of experimental animals from an ethical, social, and animal welfare-based perspective so as to obtain reliable results [113]. In fact, it has become common practice that, in order to publish scientific research, publishers request letters indicating that the research and ethics committees authorized the use of animals. The legal agreements, regulations, and guidelines for each country, as well as international standards, recommend that each study adheres to the most effective type of test and the most appropriate species for the study in order to reduce the number of animals to the bare minimum. Additionally, the use of more complex animal models, such as animals obtained *via* genetic engineering or humanized animal models, has required the expansion of these regulations.

One of the regulatory standard documents with international recognition is the Guide for the Care and Use of Laboratory Animals (NIH, Guide), which promotes the care and humane use of laboratory animals *via* a comprehensive program of publications, scientific protocols, and opinions based on the scientific experience of researchers using methodologies and practices that enable the desired results [114]. Another body handling international agreements is the Organization for Economic Cooperation and Development (OECD), which is responsible for regulating scientific protocols, tests, and analyses in order to guarantee quality results that adhere to human pathophysiology [115–119].

The implementation, development, and use of more complex animal models requiring special care will necessitate new international standards and agreements to develop better strategies and standardized protocols for scientific research. However, animal replacement is still far from becoming a viable alternative for the comparative study and development of models of human pathophysiology, at least in regard to CLD.

5. Conclusion and future outlook

Clinically speaking, the management of patients with CLD is difficult because, as mentioned above, the disease goes through several stages, each of which requires a different kind of therapeutic intervention. Clinicians and researchers still face many challenges regarding the management and study of CLD. However, there are possible ways of overcoming these challenges. More and more animal models have become available for the study of diseases, parallel to the discovery and development of new drugs. However, it is essential that we continue to improve and validate these models, particularly with regard to the molecular mechanisms that trigger and perpetuate the disease. This will ensure that they truly reflect each of the histopathological stages of human disease and will increase their predictive validity, as well as their use in the discovery of new therapeutic options.

Acknowledgements

This work was supported by the Universidad Nacional Autónoma de México (UNAM) project DGAPA-PAPIIT-IG100920 and by the Consejo Nacional de Ciencia y Tecnología (CONACYT) México through grant FORDECYT-PRONACES No. Project 74884.

Conflict of interest

The authors declare no conflict of interest.

Author details

Lourdes Rodríguez-Fragoso*, Anahí Rodríguez-López and Janet Sánchez-Quevedo
Facultad de Farmacia, Universidad Autónoma del Estado de Morelos, Cuernavaca, Mexico

*Address all correspondence to: mrodriguezf@uaem.mx

References

[1] Cheemerla S, Balakrishnan M. Global epidemiology of chronic liver disease. Clinical Liver Disease. 2021;**17**(5):365-370. DOI: 10.1002/cld.1061

[2] WHO. Global Health Estimates. Geneva: World Health Organization; 2016

[3] Sepanlou SG, Safiri S, Bisignano C. The global, regional, and national burden of cirrhosis by cause in 195 countries and territories, 1990- 2017: A systematic analysis for the Global Burden of Disease Study 2017. The Lancet. Gastroenterology & Hepatology. 2020;**5**(3):245-266. DOI: 10.1016/S2468-1253(19)30349-8

[4] Moon AM, Singal AG, Tapper EB. Contemporary epidemiology of chronic liver disease and cirrhosis. Journal of the American Gastroenterological Association. 2020;**18**(12):2650-2666. DOI: 10.1016/j.cgh.2019.07.060

[5] Asrani SK, Devarbhavi H, Eaton J, Kamath PS. Burden of liver diseases in the world. Journal of Hepatology. 2019;**70**(1):151-171. DOI: 10.1016/j.jhep.2018.09.014

[6] Chun-Chen W, Ying-Shan C, Liang C, Xin-Wen C, Meng-Ji L. Hepatitis B virus infection: Defective surface antigen expression and pathogenesis. World Journal of Gastroenterology. 2018;**24**(31):3488-3499. DOI: 10.3748/wjg.v24.i31.3488

[7] Lapa D, Garbuglia AR, Capobianchi MR, Del Porto P. Hepatitis C virus genetic variability, human immune response, and genome polymorphisms: Which is the interplay. Cell. 2019;**8**(4):305. DOI: 10.3390/cells8040305

[8] Xiao J, Wang F, Wong NK, Lv Y, Liu Y, Zhong J, et al. Epidemiological realities of alcoholic liver disease: Global burden, research trends, and therapeutic promise. Gene Expression. 2020;**20**(2):105-118. DOI: 10.3727/105221620X15952664091823

[9] Heyens LJM, Busschots D, Koek GH, Robaeys G, Francque S. Liver fibrosis in non-alcoholic fatty liver disease: From liver biopsy to non-invasive biomarkers in diagnosis and treatment. Frontiers in Medicine. 2021;**8**:615978. DOI: 10.3389/fmed.2021.615978

[10] Lapointe-Shaw L, Georgie F, Carlone D, et al. Identifying cirrhosis, decompensated cirrhosis and hepatocellular carcinoma in health administrative data: A validation study. PLoS One. 2018:13e0201120. DOI: 10.1371/journal.pone.0201120

[11] Desai AP, Mohan P, Nokes B, Sheth D, Knapp S, Boustani M, et al. Increasing economic burden in hospitalized patients with cirrhosis: Analysis of a national database. Clinical and Translational Gastroenterology. 2019;**10**:e00062. DOI: 10.14309/ctg.0000000000000062

[12] Yang JD, Hainaut P, Gores GJ, et al. A global view of hepatocellular carcinoma: Trends, risk, prevention and management. Nature Reviews. Gastroenterology & Hepatology. 2019;**16**(10):589-604. DOI: 10.1038/s41575-019-0186-y

[13] Mahmud N, Kaplan DE, Taddei TH, Goldberg DS. Incidence and mortality of acute-on-chronic liver failure using two definitions in patients with compensated cirrhosis. Hepatology. 2019;**69**:2150-2163. DOI: 10.1002/hep.30494

[14] López-Sánchez GN, Dóminguez-Pérez M, Uribe M, Nuño-Lámbarri N. The fibrogenic process and the unleashing of acute-on-chronic liver failure. Clinical and Molecular Hepatology. 2020;**26**:7-15

[15] Casulleras M, Zhang IW, López-Vicario C, Clària J. Leukocytes, systemic inflammation and immunopathology in acute-on-chronic liver failure. Cell. 2020;**9**:2632. DOI: 10.3390/cells9122632

[16] Costa D, Simbrunner B, Jachs M, Hartl L, Bauer D, Paternostro R, et al. Systemic inflammation increases across distinct stages of advanced chronic liver disease and correlates with decompensation and mortality. Journal of Hepatology. 2021;**74**:819-828. DOI: 10.1016/j.jhep.2020.10.004

[17] Zeng X, Yuan X, Cai Q, Tang C, Gao J. Circular RNA as an epigenetic regulator in chronic liver diseases. Cell. 2021;**10**(8):1945. DOI: 10.3390/cells10081945

[18] Bruneau A, Hundertmark J, Guillot A, Tacke F. Molecular and cellular mediators of the gut-liver Axis in the progression of liver diseases. Frontiers in Medicine. 2021;**8**:725390. DOI: 10.3389/fmed.2021.725390

[19] Martinou E, Pericleous M, Stefanova I, Kaur V, Angelidi AM. Diagnostic modalities of non-alcoholic fatty liver disease: From biochemical biomarkers to multi-omics non-invasive approaches. Diagnostics (Basel). 2022;**12**(2):407. DOI: 10.3390/diagnostics12020407

[20] Moura Cunha G, Navin PJ, Fowler KJ. Quantitative magnetic resonance imaging for chronic liver disease. The British journal of radiology. 2021;**94**(1121):20201377. DOI: 10.1259/bjr.20201377

[21] Singh VK, Seed TM. How necessary are animal models for modern drug discovery? Expert Opinion on Drug Discovery. 2021;**16**(12):1391-1397. DOI: 10.1080/17460441.2021.1972255

[22] McGonigle P, Ruggeri B. Animal models of human disease: Challenges in enabling translation. Biochemical Pharmacology. 2014;**87**(1):162-171. DOI: 10.1016/j.bcp.2013.08.006

[23] Tang G, Seume N, Häger C, et al. Comparing distress of mouse models for liver damage. Scientific Reports. 2020;**10**:19814. DOI: 10.1038/s41598-020-76391-w

[24] Lee SW, Kim SH, Min SO, Kim KS. Ideal experimental rat models for liver diseases. Korean journal of HBP surgery. 2011;**15**(2):67-77. DOI: 10.14701/kjhbps.2011.15.2.67

[25] Ofosu A, Ramai D, Reddy M. Non-alcoholic fatty liver disease: Controlling an emerging epidemic, challenges, and future directions. Annals of Gastroenterology. 2018;**31**(3):288-295. DOI: 10.20524/aog.2018.0240

[26] Petta S, Gastaldelli A, Rebelos E, et al. Pathophysiology of non alcoholic fatty liver disease. International Journal of Molecular Sciences. 2016;**17**:2082. DOI: 10.3390/ijms17122082

[27] Francque SM, Marchesini G, Kautz A, et al. Non-alcoholic fatty liver disease: A patient guideline. JHEP Reports: Innovation in Hepatology. 2021;**3**(5):100322. DOI: 10.1016/j.jhepr.2021.100322

[28] Savard C, Tartaglione EV, Kuver R, et al. Synergistic interaction of dietary cholesterol and dietary fat in

inducing experimental steatohepatitis. Hepatology. 2013;**57**(1):81-92. DOI: 10.1002/hep.25789

[29] Itagaki H, Shimizu K, Morikawa S. et al, Morphological and functional characterization of non-alcoholic fatty liver disease induced by a methionine-choline-deficient. International Journal of Clinical and Experimental Pathology. 2013;**6**:2683-2696

[30] Denda A, Kitayama W, Kishida H, et al. Development of hepatocellular adenomas and carcinomas associated with fibrosis in C57BL/6J male mice given a choline-deficient, Lamino acid-defined diet. Japanese Journal of Cancer Research: Gann. 2002;**93**:125-132. DOI: 10.1111/j.1349-7006.2002.tb01250.x

[31] Muriel P, López-Sánchez P, Ramos-Tovar E. Fructose and the liver. International Journal Molecular Sciences. 2021;**22**:6969

[32] Matsumoto M, Hada N, Sakamaki Y, et al. An improved mouse model that rapidly develops fibrosis in non-alcoholic steatohepatitis. International Journal of Experimental Pathology. 2013;**94**(2):93-103. DOI: 10.1111/iep.12008

[33] Lai YS, Yang TC, Chang PY, Chang SF, Ho SL, Chen HL, et al. Electronegative LDL is linked to high-fat, high-cholesterol diet induced nonalcoholic steatohepatitis in hamsters. The Journal of Nutritional Biochemistry. 2016;**30**:44-52. DOI: 10.1016/j.jnutbio.2015.11.019

[34] Tetri LH, Basaranoglu M, Brunt EM. Severe NAFLD with hepatic necroinflammatory changes in mice fed trans fats and a high-fructose corn syrup equivalent. American Journal of Physiology. Gastrointestinal and liver physiology. 2008;**295**:G987-G995. DOI: 10.1152/ajpgi.90272.2008

[35] Min HK, Kapoor A, Fuchs M, et al. Increased hepatic synthesis and desregulation of cholesterol metabolism is associated with the severity of nonalcoholic fatty liver disease. Cell Metabolism. 2012;**15**(5):665-674. DOI: 10.1016/j.cmet.2012.04.004

[36] Wortham M, He L, Gyamfi M. The transition from fatty liver to NASH associates with SAMe depletion in db/db mice fed a methionine choline-deficient diet. Digestive Diseases and Sciences. 2008;**53**(10):2761-2774. DOI: 10.1007/s10620-007-0193-7

[37] Carmiel-Haggai M, Cederbaum AI, Nieto N. A high-fat diet leads to the progression of non-alcoholic fatty liver disease in obese rats. The FASEB Journal. 2005;**19**(1):136-138. DOI: 10.1096/fj.04-2291fje

[38] Domenicali M, Caraceni P, Giannone F, et al. A novel model of CCl4-induced cirrhosis with ascites in the mouse. Journal of Hepatology. 2009;**51**:991-999. DOI: 10.1016/j.jhep.2009.09.008

[39] Fortea JI, Fernández-Mena C, Puerto M, et al. Comparison of two protocols of carbon tetrachloride-induced cirrhosis in rats—Improving yield and reproducibility. Scientific Reports. 2018;**8**:1-10. DOI: 10.1038/s41598-018-27427-9

[40] Wallace MC, Hamesch K, Lunova M, et al. Standard operating procedures in experimental liver research: Thioacetamide model in mice and rats. Laboratory Animals. 2015;**49**:21-29. DOI: 10.1177/0023677215573040

[41] Bona S, Moreira AJ, Rodrigues GR, et al. Diethylnitrosamine-induced

cirrhosis in Wistar rats: An experimental feasibility study. Protoplasma. 2015;**252**:825-833. DOI: 10.1007/s00709-014-0719-8

[42] Wang PW, Hung YC, Li WT, et al. Systematic revelation of the protective effect and mechanism of Cordycep sinensis on diethylnitrosamine-induced rat hepatocellular carcinoma with proteomics. Oncotarget. 2016;7:60270-60289. DOI: 10.18632/oncotarget.11201

[43] Chen YJ, Wallig MA, Jeffery EH. Dietary broccoli lessens development of fatty liver and liver cancer in mice given diethylnitrosamine and fed a Western or control diet. The Journal of Nutrition. 2016;**146**(3):542-550. DOI: 10.3945/jn.115.228148

[44] Gao J, Xiong R, Xiong D, et al. The adenosine monophosphate (AMP) analog, 5-aminoimidazole-4-carboxamide ribonucleotide (AICAR) inhibits HEPATOSTEATOSIS and liver tumorigenesis in a high-fat diet murine model treated with diethylnitrosamine (DEN). Medical Science Monitor: International Medical Journal of Experimental and Clinical Research. 2018;**24**:8533-8543. DOI: 10.12659/MSM.910544

[45] Solt DB, Cayama E, Tsuda H, et al. Promotion of liver cancer development by brief exposure to dietary 2-acetylaminofluorene plus partial hepatectomy or carbon tetrachloride. Cancer Research. 1983;**43**:188-191

[46] Kountouras J, Billing BH. Scheuer PJ, Prolonged bile duct obstruction: A new experimental model for cirrhosis in the rat. British Journal of Experimental Pathology. 1984;**65**:305-311

[47] Perfield JW 2nd, Ortinau LC, Pickering RT, et al. Altered hepatic lipid metabolism contributes to nonalcoholic fatty liver disease in leptin-deficient Ob/Ob mice. Journal of Obesity. 2013;**2013**:296537. DOI: 10.1155/2013/296537

[48] Opazo-Ríos L, Soto-Catalán M, Lázaro I, et al. Meta-inflammation and de novo lipogenesis markers are involved in metabolic associated fatty liver disease progression in BTBR Ob/Ob mice. International Journal of Molecular Sciences. 2022;**23**(7):3965. DOI: 10.3390/ijms23073965

[49] Kim K, Jung Y, Min S, et al. Caloric restriction of db/db mice reverts hepatic steatosis and body weight with divergent hepatic metabolism. Scientific Reports. 2016;**6**:30111. DOI: 10.1038/srep30111

[50] Palladini G, Ferrigno A, Di Pasqua LG, et al. Associations between serum trace elements and inflammation in two animal models of nonalcoholic fatty liver disease. PLoS One. 2020;**15**(12):e0243179. DOI: 10.1371/journal.pone.0243179

[51] Teixeira de Lemos E, Reis F, Baptista S, et al. Exercise training decreases proinflammatory profile in Zucker diabetic (type 2) fatty rats. Nutrition. 2009;**25**:330-339. DOI: 10.1016/j.nut.2008.08.014

[52] Moslehi A, Hamidi-Zad Z. Role of SREBPs in liver diseases: A mini-review. Journal of Clinical and Translational Hepatology. 2018;**6**(3):332-338. DOI: 10.14218/JCTH.2017.00061

[53] Willebrords J, Alves Pereira IV, Maes M, et al. Strategies, models and biomarkers in experimental non-alcoholic fatty liver disease research. Progress in Lipid Research. 2015;**59**:106-125. DOI: 10.1016/j.plipres.2015.05.002

[54] Goto T, Lee JY, Teraminami A, et al. Activation of peroxisome proliferator-activated receptor-alpha stimulates both differentiation and fatty acid oxidation in adipocytes. Journal of Lipid Research. 2011;**52**:873-884. DOI: 10.1194/jlr.M011320

[55] Aller MA, Lorente L, Alonso S, Arias J. A model of cholestasis in the rat, using a microsurgical technique. Scandinavian Journal of Gastroenterology. 1993;**28**: 10-14. DOI: 10.3109/00365529309096038

[56] Liu XH, Chen Y, Wang TL, et al. Establishment of a D-galactosamine/ Lipopolysaccharide induced acute-on-chronic liver failure model in rats. Chinese Journal of Hepatology. 1993;**15**:771-775

[57] Romualdo GR, Leroy K, Costa CJS, et al. In vivo and In vitro models of hepatocellular carcinoma: Current strategies for translational modeling. Cancers. 2021;**13**:5583. DOI: 10.3390/ cancers13215583

[58] Juanola O, Martínez-López S, Francés R, Gómez-Hurtado I. Non-alcoholic fatty liver disease: Metabolic, genetic, epigenetic and environmental risk factors. International Journal of Environmental Research and Public Health. 2021;**18**(10):5227. DOI: 10.3390/ ijerph18105227

[59] Geier A, Tiniakos D, Denk H, Trauner M. From the origin of NASH to the future of metabolic fatty liver disease. Gut. 2021;**70**(8):1570-1579. DOI: 10.1136/gutjnl-2020-323202

[60] Mota M, Banini BA, Cazanave SC, Sanyal AJ. Molecular mechanisms of lipotoxicity and glucotoxicity in nonalcoholic fatty liver disease. Metabolism. 2016;**65**:1049-1061. DOI: 10.1016/j.metabol.2016.02.014

[61] Marra F, Svegliati-Baroni G. Lipotoxicity and the gut-liver axis in NASH pathogenesis. Journal of Hepatology. 2018;**68**:280-295. DOI: 10.1016/j.jhep.2017.11.014

[62] Mihm S. Danger-associated molecular patterns (DAMPs): Molecular triggers for sterile inflammation in the liver. International Journal of Molecular Sciences. 2018;**19**:3104. DOI: 10.3390/ ijms19103104

[63] Buzzetti E, Pinzani M, Tsochatzis EA. The multiple-hit pathogenesis of non-alcoholic fatty liver disease (NAFLD). Metabolism, Clinical and Experimental. 2016;**65**:1038-1048. DOI: 10.1016/j.metabol.2015.12.012

[64] Gadd VL, Skoien R, Powell EE, et al. The portal inflammatory infiltrate and ductular reaction in human nonalcoholic fatty liver disease. Hepatology. 2014;**59**:1393-1405. DOI: 10.1002/ hep.26937

[65] Olsen AL, Bloomer SA, Chan EP, et al. Hepatic stellate cells require a stiff environment for myofibroblastic differentiation. American Journal of Physiology, Gastrointestinal and liver physiology. 2011;**302**:G110-G118. DOI: 10.1152/ajpgi.00412.2010

[66] Moran-Salvador E, Mann J. Epigenetics and liver fibrosis. Cellular and Molecular Gastroenterology and Hepatology. 2017;**4**:125-134. DOI: 10.1016/j.jcmgh.2017.04.007

[67] Miao CG, Yang YY, He X, et al. Wnt signaling in liver fibrosis: Progress, challenges and potential directions. Biochimie. 2013;**95**:2326-2335. DOI: 10.1016/j.biochi.2013.09.003

[68] Elpek GÖ. Cellular and molecular mechanisms in the pathogenesis of liver fibrosis: An update. World Journal of

Gastroenterology. 2014;**20**:7260-7276. DOI: 10.3748/wjg.v20.i23.7260

[69] Dewidar B, Meyer C, Dooley S, Meindl-Beinker AN. TGF-β in hepatic stellate cell activation and liver fibrogenesis-updated 2019. Cell. 2019;**8**:1419. DOI: 10.3390/cells8111419

[70] Kohli R, Kirby M, Xanthakos SA, et al. High-fructose, medium chain trans fat diet induces liver fibrosis and elevates plasma coenzyme Q9 in a novel murine model of obesity and nonalcoholic steatohepatitis. Hepatology. 2010;**52**:934-944. DOI: 10.1002/hep.23797

[71] Ipsen DH, Lykkesfeldt J, Tveden-Nyborg P. Animal models of fibrosis in nonalcoholic steatohepatitis: Do they reflect human disease? Advances in Nutrition. 2020;**11**:1696-1711. DOI: 10.1093/advances/nmaa081

[72] Ramadori P, Weiskirchen R, Trebicka J, Streetz K. Mouse models of metabolic liver injury. Laboratory Animals. 2015;**49**:47-58. DOI: 10.1177/0023677215570078

[73] Rives C, Fougerat A, Ellero-Simatos S, et al. Oxidative stress in NAFLD: Role of nutrients and food contaminants. Biomolecules. 2020;**10**(12):1702. DOI: 10.3390/biom10121702

[74] Boland ML, Oró D, Tølbøl KS, et al. Towards a standard diet-induced and biopsy-confirmed mouse model of non-alcoholic steatohepatitis: Impact of dietary fat source. World Journal of Gastroenterology. 2019;**25**(33):4904-4920. DOI: 10.3748/wjg.v25.i33.4904

[75] Charlton M, Krishnan A, Viker K, et al. Fast food diet mouse: Novel small animal model of NASH with ballooning, progressive fibrosis, and high physiological fidelity to the human condition. American Journal of Physiology. Gastrointestinal and Liver Physiology. 2011;**301**(5):G825-G834. DOI: 10.1152/ajpgi.00145.2011

[76] Cremonese C, Schierwagen R, Uschner FE, et al. Short-term Western diet aggravates non-alcoholic fatty liver disease (NAFLD) with portal hypertension in TGR(mREN2)27 rats. International Journal of Molecular Sciences. 2020;**21**(9):3308. DOI: 10.3390/ijms21093308

[77] Peng C, Stewart AG, Woodman OL, et al. Non-alcoholic steatohepatitis: A review of its mechanism, models and medical treatments. Frontiers in Pharmacology. 2020;**11**:603926. DOI: 10.3389/fphar.2020.603926

[78] Kořínková L, Pražienková V, Černá L, et al. Pathophysiology of NAFLD and NASH in experimental models: The role of food intake regulating peptides. Frontiers in Endocrinology. 2020;**11**:597583. DOI: 10.3389/fendo.2020.597583

[79] Shimomura I, Bashmakov Y, Horton JD. Increased levels of nuclear SREBP-1c associated with fatty livers in two mouse models of diabetes mellitus. The Journal of Biological Chemistry. 1999;**274**(42):30028-300032. DOI: 10.1074/jbc.274.42.30028

[80] Leff T, Mathews ST, Camp HS. Review: Peroxisome proliferator-activated receptor-γ and its role in the development and treatment of diabetes. Experimental Diabesity Research. 2004;**5**(2):99-109. DOI: 10.1080/15438600490451668

[81] Ramon S, Bancos S, Thatcher TH, et al. Peroxisome proliferator-activated receptor γ B cell-specific–deficient

mice have an impaired antibody response. Journal of Immunology. 2012;**189**(10):4740-4747. DOI: 10.4049/jimmunol.1200956

[82] Kanda T, Goto T, Hirotsu Y. Molecular mechanisms driving progression of liver cirrhosis towards hepatocellular carcinoma in chronic hepatitis B and C infections: A review. International Journal of Molecular Sciences. 2019;**20**(6):1358. DOI: 10.3390/ijms20061358

[83] Gustot T, Moreau R. Acute-on-chronic liver failure vs. traditional acute decompensation of cirrhosis. Journal of Hepatology. 2018;**69**:1384-1393. DOI: 10.1016/j.jhep.2018.08.024

[84] Molina-Sánchez P, Lujambio A. Experimental models for preclinical research in hepatocellular carcinoma. In: Hoshida Y, editor. Hepatocellular Carcinoma: Translational Precision Medicine Approaches. Humana Press; 2019. pp. 333-358. DOI: 10.1007/978-3-030-21540-8_16

[85] Llovet JM, Zucman-Rossi J, Pikarsky E, et al. Hepatocellular carcinoma. Disease Primers. 2016;**2**:16018. DOI: 10.1038/nrdp.2016.18

[86] Shibata T, Aburatani H. Exploration of liver cancer genomes. Nature Reviews. Gastroenterology & Hepatology. 2014;**11**:340-349. DOI: 10.1038/nrgastro.2014.6

[87] Kemelo MK, Wojnarová L, Kutinová Canová N, Farghali H. D-galactosamine/lipopolysaccharide-induced hepatotoxicity downregulates sirtuin 1 in rat liver: Role of sirtuin 1 modulation in hepatoprotection. Physiological Research. 2014;**63**:615-623. DOI: 10.33549/physiolres.932761

[88] Arroyo V, García-Martinez R, Salvatella X. Human serum albumin, systemic inflammation, and cirrhosis. Journal of Hepatology. 2014;**61**:396-407. DOI: 10.1016/j.jhep.2014.04.012

[89] Yang F, Li X, Wang LK, Wang LW, Han XQ, Zhang H, et al. Inhibitions of NF-κB and TNF-α result in differential effects in rats with acute on chronic liver failure induced by d-Gal and LPS. Inflammation. 2014;**37**(3):848-857. DOI: 10.1007/s10753-013-9805-x

[90] Aitio A, Aitio ML, Camus AM, et al. Cytochrome P-450 isozyme pattern is related to individual susceptibility to diethylnitrosamine-induced liver cancer in rats. Japanese Journal of Cancer Research. 1991;**82**(2):146-156. DOI: 10.1111/j.1349-7006.1991.tb01822.x

[91] Connor F, Rayner TF, Aitken SJ, et al. Mutational landscape of a chemically induced mouse model of liver cancer. Journal of Hepatology. 2018;**69**(4):840-850. DOI: 10.1016/j.jhep.2018.06.009

[92] Kushida M, Kamendulis LM, Peat TJ, Klaunig JE. Dose-related induction of hepatic preneoplastic lesions by diethylnitrosamine in C57BL/6 mice. Toxicologic Pathology 2011;**39**(5):776-786. DOI:10.1177/0192623311409596

[93] Uehara T, Ainslie GR, Kutanzi K, et al. Molecular mechanisms of fibrosis-associated promotion of liver carcinogenesis. Toxicological Sciences. 2013;**132**:53-63. DOI: 10.1093/toxsci/kfs342

[94] Memon A, Pyao Y, Jung Y, et al. A modified protocol of diethylnitrosamine administration in mice to model hepatocellular carcinoma. International Journal of Molecular Sciences. 2020;**21**(15):5461. DOI: 10.3390/ijms21155461

[95] Uehara T, Pogribny IP, Rusyn I. The DEN and CCl4-induced mouse model of fibrosis and inflammation-associated hepatocellular carcinoma. Current Protocols in Pharmacology. 2014;**66**:30

[96] Kurma K, Manches O, Chuffart F, et al. DEN-induced rat model reproduces key features of human hepatocellular carcinoma. Cancers. 2021;**13**(19):4981. DOI: 10.3390/cancers13194981

[97] Lee G. Review article: Paradoxical effects of phenobarbital on mouse hepatocarcinogenesis. Toxicologic Pathology. 2000;**28**:215-225. DOI: 10.1177/019262330002800201

[98] Romualdo GR, Grassi TF, Goto RL, et al. An integrative analysis of chemically-induced cirrhosis-associated hepatocarcinogenesis: Histological, biochemical and molecular features. Toxicology Letters. 2017;**281**:84-94. DOI: 10.1016/j.toxlet.2017.09.015

[99] Pereira MA, Herren-Freund SL, Long RE. Dose-response relationship of phenobarbital promotion of diethylnitrosamine initiated tumors in rat liver. Cancer Letters. 1986;**32**:305-311. DOI: 10.1016/0304-3835(86)90183-7

[100] Yu DY, Moon HB, Son JK, et al. Incidence of hepatocellular carcinoma in transgenic mice expressing the hepatitis B virus X-protein. Journal of Hepatology. 1999;**31**:123-132. DOI: 10.1016/s0168-8278(99)80172-x

[101] Lai MW, Liang KH, Lin WR, et al. Hepatocarcinogenesis in transgenic mice carrying hepatitis B virus pre-S/S gene with the sW172* mutation. Oncogene. 2016;**5**:e273. DOI: 10.1038/oncsis.2016.77

[102] Verma B, Wesa A. Establishment of humanized mice from peripheral blood mononuclear cells or cord blood CD34+ hematopoietic stem cells for immune-oncology studies evaluating new therapeutic agents. Current Protocols in Pharmacology. 2020;**89**: 1-19. DOI: 10.1002/cpph.77

[103] Walsh NC, Kenney LL, Jangalwe S, et al. Humanized mouse models of clinical disease. Annual Review of Pathology. 2017;**12**:187-215. DOI: 10.1146/annurev-pathol-052016-100332

[104] Robinson NB, Krieger K, Khan FM, et al. The current state of animal models in research: A review. International Journal of Surgery (London, England). 2019;**72**:9-13. DOI: 10.1016/j.ijsu.2019.10.015

[105] Tsukamoto H, Matsuoka M, French SW. Experimental models of hepatic fibrosis: A review. Seminars in Liver Disease. 1990;**10**(1):56-65. DOI: 10.1055/s-2008-1040457

[106] Popov Y, Schuppan D. Targeting liver fibrosis: Strategies for development and validation of antifibrotic therapies. Hepatology (Baltimore, Md.). 2009;**50**(4):1294-1306. DOI: 10.1002/hep.23123

[107] Land WG. Cell-autonomous (cell intrinsic) stress responses. Damage-Associated Molecular Patterns in Human Diseases. 2018;**28**:377-426. DOI: 10.1007/978-3-319-78655-1_18

[108] Sensini F, Inta D, Palme R, et al. The impact of handling technique and handling frequency on laboratory mouse welfare is sex-specific. Scientific Reports. 2020;**10**:17281. DOI: 10.1038/s41598-020-74279-3

[109] Official Journal of the European Union. Directive 2010/63/EU of the European Parliament and of the Council on the protection of animals used for scientific purposes. 2010. L276/33–L276/79 (22 September 2010). [website].

Available from: http://eurlex.europa.eu/LexUriServ/LexUriServ.do?uri=OJ:L:2010:276:0033:0079:en:PDF.

[110] Hendriksen CF. The ethics of research involving animals: A review of the Nuffield Council on Bioethics report from a three Rs perspective. Alternatives to laboratory animals: ATLA. 2005;**33**(6):659-662. DOI: 10.1177/026119290503300604

[111] American Association for Laboratory Animal Science (AALAS). Cost of Caring: Recognizing Human Emotions in the Care of Laboratory Animals. Memphis, TN: AALAS; 2001

[112] Medina LV. Building a Culture of Animal Welfare: Past, Present and Future. São Paulo: Abbott Laboratories; 2008. DOI: 10.5016/1806-8774.2008.v10pT104

[113] Kilkenny C, Browne WJ, Cuthill IC. Improving bioscience research reporting: The ARRIVE guidelines for reporting animal research. Veterinary Clinical Pathology. 2012;**41**(1):27-31. DOI: 10.1111/j.1939-165X.2012.00418.x

[114] National Research Council (US) Committee for the Update of the Guide for the Care and Use of Laboratory Animals. Guide for the Care and Use of Laboratory Animals. 8th ed. Washington (DC): National Academies Press (US); 2011

[115] Gordon K. The OECD Guidelines and Other Corporate Responsibility Instruments: A Comparison, OECD Working Papers on International Investment, 2001/05, OECD; 2001. [website]. Publishing. DOI: 10.1787/302255465771

[116] Liebsch M, Spielmann H. Currently available in vitro methods used in the regulatory toxicology. Toxicology Letters. 2002;**127**(1-3):127-134. DOI: 10.1016/s0378-4274(01)00492-1

[117] Organization for Economic Co-operation and Development (OECD). 1983. OECD Publications Office, Paris, France

[118] Organization for Economic Co-operation and Development (OECD). Final Report of the OECD Workshop on Harmonization of Validation and Acceptance Criteria for Alternative Toxicological Tests Methods. Paris, France: OECD Publications Office; 1996

[119] Brown MJ, Symonowicz C, Medina LV, et al. Culture of care: Organizational responsibilities. In: Weichbrod RH, Thompson GAH, Norton JN, editors. Management of Animal Care and Use Programs in Research, Education, and Testing. 2nd ed. Boca Raton (FL): CRC Press/Taylor & Francis; 2018

Chapter 4

Survival Fate of Hepatic Stem/Progenitor and Immune Cells in a Liver Fibrosis/Cirrhosis Animal Model and Clinical Implications

Min Yan, Deyu Hu, Zhenyu Wu, Jiejuan Lai, Leida Zhang, Hongyu Zhang, Sijin Li and Lianhua Bai

Abstract

This chapter provides novel information about the survival features of hepatic resident stem/progenitor cells ($NG2^+$ HSPs) during liver fibrosis/cirrhotic development. A well-defined diethylnitrosamine (DEN)-induced liver fibrosis/cirrhotic/cancer mouse model was developed to evaluate the fate of the HSPs and its clinical implications. This model possess three time-zones during the disease development: fibrosis (3–5 weeks post-DEN), cirrhosis (6–10 weeks post-DEN), and cancers (up to 10 weeks post-DEN). During this process, the model represents histological patterns similar to those described in humans and shows better survival of the HSPs in the fibrotic zone, which was correlated with inflammatory signals, as compared to the cirrhotic zone. It has also been discovered that immune $CD8^+$ T cells in the fibrotic zone are beneficial in liver fibrosis resolution, suggesting that the fibrotic time zone is important for mobilizing endogenous HSPs and cell-based therapy. As such, we hypothesize that clinical strategies in fibrotic/cirrhotic liver treatment are necessary either in time at the fibrotic phase or to adopt an approach of regulating HSP viability when the disease develops into the cirrhotic phase.

Keywords: apoptosis, diethylnitrosamine, hepatic stem/progenitor cells, inflammation, liver fibrosis/cirrhosis, proliferation

1. Introduction

The healthy liver performs over 500 different functions to maintain its homeostasis [1, 2], and any assault could not only impact the architecture of hepatic cells [3] but also injure niche cells, like inflammatory and immune cells such as CD8-positive cytotoxic T lymphocyte subset ($CD8^+$ T cells) which have been recently highlighted [4]. Liver cirrhosis is an end-stage liver disease (ESLD) and a major cause of morbidity and mortality globally [5]. It is often caused by acute liver injury or the progressive development of liver fibrosis or other chronic liver disease such as virus infection, etc. In China, the total number of patients with various types of chronic liver disease exceeds

300 million, and more than 1 million people die each year from ESLD [6]. According to the Centers for Disease Control (CDC), ESLD is the twelfth leading cause of death in the United States, with approximately 44,000 deaths per year [7]. For example, chronic hepatitis B virus (HBV) infection-mediated ESLD and inflammatory disease are global public health issues. It was estimated in 2017 that 257 million people live with chronic HBV infection, a prevalence of 3.5% [8], and there are 93 million people infected with HBV living in China [9]. Approximately 15–40% of patients with chronic HBV will develop liver cirrhosis, and 4–5% of patients may progress toward decompensated liver cirrhosis (DLC) [9], denoted in the chemical reagent diethylnitrosamine (DEN)-induced liver fibrosis/cirrhosis animal model at 6–10 weeks post-DEN in this chapter [9]. The 5-year mortality in patients with compensated liver cirrhosis (CLC), denoted as fibrotic phase (6–10 weeks post-DEN) in this chapter, is 14–20% and with DLC as high as 70–86% [5, 8, 9] which imposes a substantial health burden on many countries. It has been studied in animals that continuous activation of hepatic stellate cells (HSCs) leading to accumulation and over-deposition of the extracellular matrix (ECM) in the parenchymal liver compartment [10, 11] is a key mechanism for the liver from homeostasis to fibrosis (3–5 weeks post-DEN) to cirrhosis (6–10 weeks post-DEN) and eventually the outcomes of liver cancer like hepatocyte cellular carcinoma (HCC, >10 weeks post-DEN), which is the most common liver cancer (**Figure 1A**). In humans, there are generally four categories from healthy liver to HCC, including homeostasis, compensation liver cirrhosis phase (CLC), decompensation liver cirrhosis phase (DLC), and liver cancer (HCC) (**Figure 1A**). Of note, there are currently none of available treatments to specifically target other than liver transplantation. Unfortunately, there are simply not enough donated livers to meet the demands; therefore, research on nonsurgical strategies to prevent the development of chronic liver disease is urgently needed. Stem cell therapy is one of the options for treating liver fibrosis/cirrhosis [12] and can partially recover liver function [13, 14]. However, the problem is that clinical trials using stem cells to treat liver fibrosis/cirrhosis, especially for DLC treatment, seem not to be so successful [12, 15–17] because of the short-term survival of cells in DLC microenvironment [18].

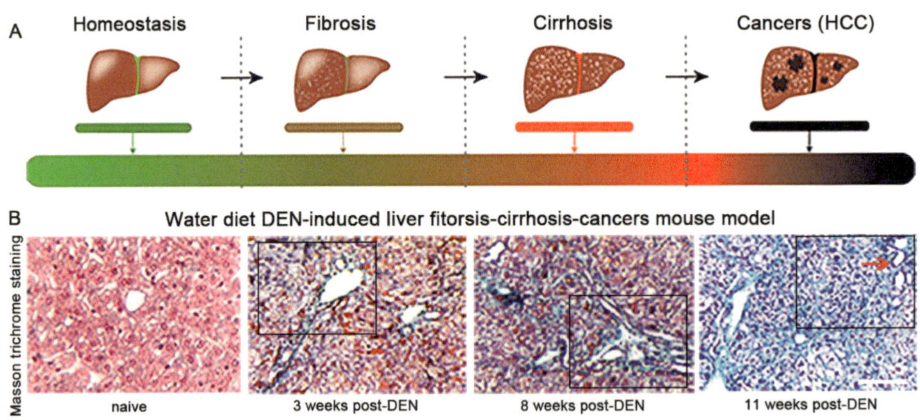

Figure 1.
Application of DEN produces a relatively sharp line in different phases during the model disease development. (A) Evolution of ESLD during disease development. (B) Masson trichrome staining identified pathogenesis (blue, boxes) in hepatic sections at different phases of DEN-induced liver fibrosis-cirrhosis-cancers (HCC, an arrow) in a mouse model. Scale bar = 100 μm.

Therefore, if animal models with liver fibrosis/cirrhosis laboratory scores capture patients with the same disease, pathological features would be very meaningful for future clinical stem cell-based therapeutic strategies. As such, we have for the first time successfully set up a liver fibrosis/cirrhosis/cancer animal model in C57BL/6 mice in 2015, demonstrating histological patterns similar to those described in humans during the disease process [19]. Interestingly, this model shows that during the disease process, the resident HSPs (denoted as $NG2^+$ HSPs) [18] respond to DEN-mediated inflammatory signals differently, resulting in different fates during liver fibrosis/cirrhosis development. More interestingly, immune $CD8^+$ T cells have also been found recently to involve in improving liver fibrotic load [20]. In this chapter, we have provided novel information on the correlation of hepatic inflammatory activity with microenvironment resident HSPs ($NG2^+$ HSPs) and how HSP survival fate are also related to the hepatic resident $CD8^+$ T cells during the disease development on this model.

2. The chemical reagent (DEN)-induced liver fibrosis/cirrhosis and carcinogenesis in C57BL/6 inbred mice fed a drinking water diet

DEN is a nitrosamine-containing chemical reagent, and its toxic properties in mammals are well established [21–23]. Studies have shown that oral administration of the smallest quantities of DEN or dimethylnitrosamine (DMN) results in severe hepatic cell injury in both animals and humans [24–27]. The most prominent chemical reagents are intense neutrophilic infiltration, extensive centrilobular hemorrhagic necrosis, bile duct proliferation, fibrosis, and bridging necrosis that end in hepatocarcinogenesis [28].

DEN was first brought to general attention in 1937 [29] when it was reported to be the causative agent that induces liver injury in men. This assumption was experimentally confirmed in 1954 by Barnes and Magee, who found that a single oral or parental dose (20–40 mg/kg body weight) of the reagent acts primarily as a liver poison producing severe liver necrosis in both small and large animals [30] of which the landmark experiment shows a sharp line of demarcation between the totally destroyed parenchyma and apparently uninjured liver cell areas in the model liver lesions [30]. Furthermore, the animal model shows that chronic application of the chemical agent in rats resulted in a high incidence of hepatic malignancy [31]. The extension of these studies has been subsequently revealed by many other researchers [30, 32, 33]. These findings suggest that the chemical and physical properties of DEN may be of interest for understanding the hepatic pathological characteristics underlying the evolution of liver fibrosis/cirrhosis/HCC formation [25], although the hepatotoxic and carcinogenic mechanism was not known until 1963 [34].

Moreover, although the application of DEN has become a well-established model in animals for studies of the pathogenetic alterations underlying the formation of liver fibrosis, cirrhosis and cancers, the single diet DEN for analyzing liver fibrosis/cirrhosis in wild-type mice has never been investigated. As such, applied C57BL/6 wild-type inbred mice with a single diet of 0.014% DEN in drinking water; 6 days/week for 15 weeks, we successfully induced a liver fibrosis/cirrhosis/cancer mouse model [19]. The model shows that DEN is extremely effective in inducing hepatic fibrosis [21], cirrhosis and cancers (**Figure 1B**) that are compatible with the deterioration of liver functions [22, 35].

3. Prolonged single-diet DEN administration within drinking water in C57BL/6 mice results in hepatic inflammation that impacts resident HSP fate

At present, although stem cell-based therapy as an emerging approach is widely studied for a variety of causes of CLF and CLC, for example, nonalcoholic fatty liver disease (NAFLD) [36], alcohol-associated liver disease (ALD) [37], and drug-induced liver injury (DILI) [38] etc.; however, due to the short-term survival of HSPs in the cirrhotic niche [18], the effect seems not to be so successful in the clinic.

It is known that inflammation is involved in pathological features during regenerative fibrotic nodule formation, which replaces normal functional liver parenchyma to remodel the vasculature in the liver and ultimately compromises liver function [39–42]. Histologically, the inflammatory responses to toxic signals of DEN and influence fibrotic load have been characterized by our [18] and other studies [43]. These

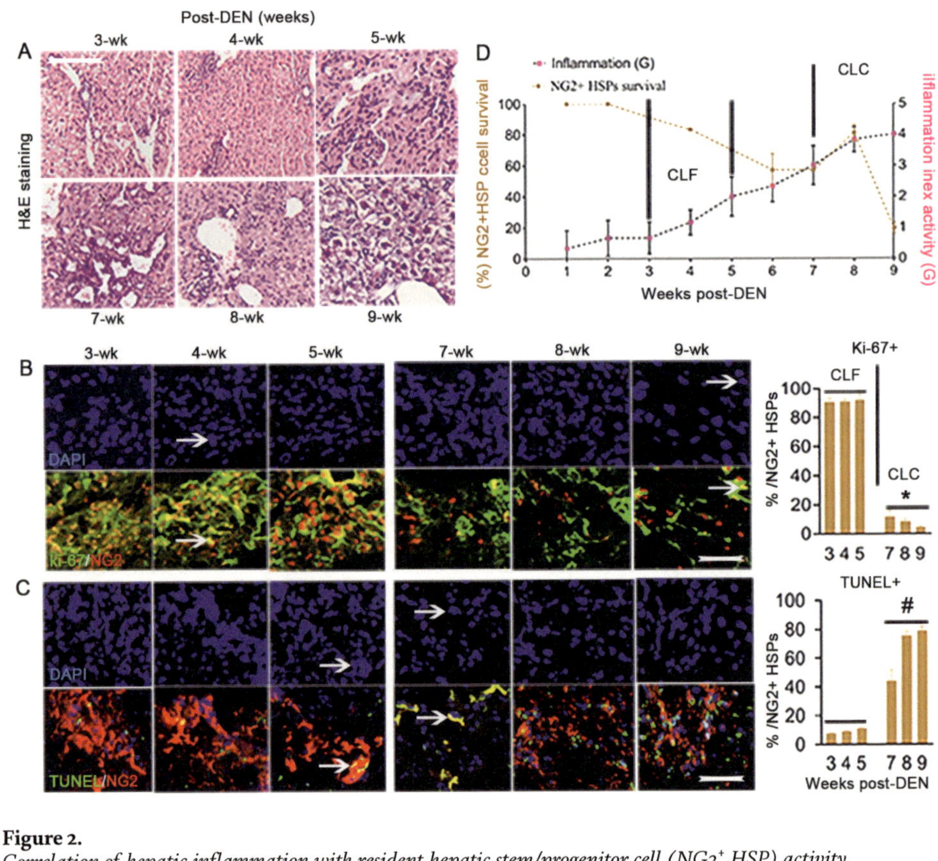

Figure 2.
Correlation of hepatic inflammation with resident hepatic stem/progenitor cell (NG2⁺ HSP) activity.
(A) H&E staining detected hepatic infiltrating mononuclear cells at the fibrotic phase (3–5 weeks post-DEN) and cirrhotic phase (7–9 weeks post-DEN) during DEN-induced liver development. Scale bar = 100 μm.
(B) Using anti-NG2 (red) and Ki-67 (green) antibodies for hepatic resident $NG2^+$ HSP cell proliferation at the fibrotic phase (3–5 weeks post-DEN) and cirrhotic phase (7–9 weeks post-DEN) (merged as brown, arrows) during DEN-induced liver development. Scale bar = 200 μm. (C) The TUNEL (green) assay identified hepatic resident $NG2^+$ HSP cell (red) apoptosis (merged as brown, arrows) at the fibrotic phase (3–5 weeks post-DEN) and cirrhotic phase (7–9 weeks post-DEN) during DEN-induced liver development. Scale bar = 200 μm.
(D) The International Simplified Grading and Staging System (ISGSS) was used for inflammation index activity and immunofluorescence staining for inflammation degree (denoted as G, pink) and $NG2^+$ HSP activity (brown) evaluation. $^{\#}p < 0.05$ *vs. fibrotic phase, with Student's t test.*

studies exhibit monocyte infiltration and collagen deposition accompanies varying degrees of deformation of liver structures identified by hematoxylin-eosin (H&E) and Masson's trichrome staining, resulting in aggravated fiber load. Advanced fibrosis of the liver has been considered irreversible and is itself a risk factor for liver cancers such as HCC. Traditionally, it has often been thought that a beneficial way to prevent advanced fibrosis or liver cirrhosis is to control inflammation, while a recent study suggests that inflammation may be helpful for resident HSP activation and survival during hepatic disease development [18].

Several strategies to mobilize endogenous HSP-based therapies have been studied within the past few decades, but the underlying relationship between the HSP cells with their inflammatory niche signals in injured liver is largely unknown. We have currently demonstrated that prolonged oral water feeding with 0.014% DEN produces a sharp line between liver fibrosis (3–5 weeks post-DEN) and cirrhosis cancers (6–10 weeks post-DEN) [18]. Of note, in this model, we have found an interesting phenomenon, showing a positive correlation of resident HSP ($NG2^+$ HSP) survival with hepatic inflammation in the fibrotic stage (3–5 weeks post-DEN) and when an irregular inflammatory response occurred in the later fibrosis or cirrhosis stage (3–5 weeks post-DEN), the HSP cells ($NG2^+$ HSPs) died rapidly (**Figure 2A** and **D**), represented as gradually reduced Ki-67^+ cells of $NG2^+$ HSPs (**Figure 2B**) and increased terminal deoxynucleotidyl transferase (TdT) dUTP Nick-End Labeling (TUNEL)-expression within the $NG2^+$ HSPs (**Figure 2C**), suggesting that some unknown signals in the cirrhotic liver niche could trigger the HSP cell ($NG2^+$ HSP) apoptosis [44].

4. The 0.014% DEN-treated liver fibrosis/cirrhosis mouse model-associated immune role of resident hepatic $CD8^+$ T cells

The DEN-induced dynamic liver disease mouse model lining hepatic homeostasis, fibrosis, cirrhotic and HCC phases seems similar to humans. Clinically, liver cirrhosis comprises two stages as abovementioned: the fibrotic phase, often asymptomatic, also known as a compensated stage (CLC), and the cirrhotic phase or decompensated stage, characterized by complications arising from portal hypertension and hepatic insufficiency (DLC) [45, 46]. The DLC is also considered a systemic disease because it affects most organs and systems of the body, including the immune system [47, 48].

On the topic of fibrotic/cirrhotic liver disease and immune correlation, we would like to mention the latest idea termed cirrhosis-associated immune dysfunction (CAID) [49, 50], characterized by two key components: systemic inflammation and immune deficiency. It shows variable intensity depending on the stage of liver fibrosis/cirrhosis and the presence of incidental events. With this, we would like to give a better representative example of cirrhosis-mediated liver failure, acute-on-chronic liver failure (ACLF), a syndrome characterized by acute decompensation of cirrhosis, hepatic and/or extrahepatic organ failures and high short-term mortality [51], as well as the most severe immune alterations in the patients with this disease [51]. Patients with liver cirrhosis who develop these stages/diseases combine the highest grade of systemic inflammation [41] and severe immunodeficiency [52], which leads not only to an increased risk of infections but also to pathogenic liver organ failure [53] or cancers (HCC) [54, 55]; however, how these phenomena underlie biological substrates is unclear. One study shows for the first time that depression or anxiety grade of patients with liver cirrhosis is correlated with $CD8^+$ T-cell signs [56], suggesting that

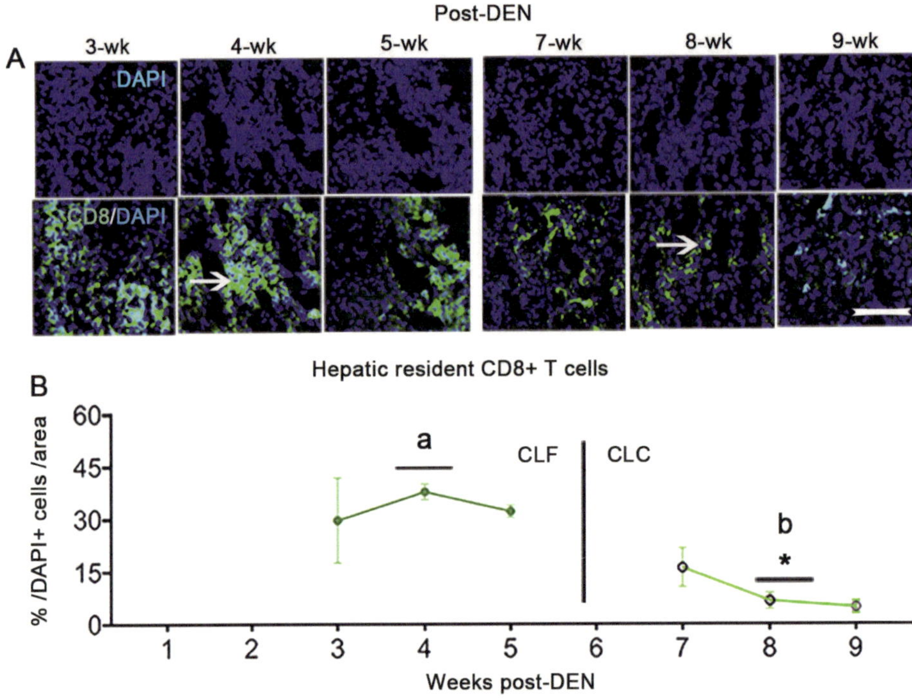

Figure 3.
Dynamic changes in hepatic resident CD8⁺ T cells during DEN-induced liver fibrosis/cirrhosis development. (A) The expression of hepatic resident CD8⁺ T cells was higher in the fibrotic phase (3–5 weeks post-DEN) than in the cirrhotic phase (7–9 weeks post-DEN). Scale bar = 200 μm. (Ba, b) Hepatic resident CD8⁺ T cells dramatically increased at 4 weeks post-DEN (a) and sharply decreased at 8 weeks post-DEN (b) during model disease development. $^{*}p < 0.05$, *8 vs. 4 weeks, with Student's t test.*

an imbalance of CD8⁺ T cells may be a factor facilitating neurological disease patients with cirrhotic liver disease.

Although at present it is considered that advanced liver fibrosis to be irreversible, recent clinical evidence demonstrating substantial fibrosis resolution following different successful treatments overturned this dogma [57]. Accordingly, significant efforts have been made to inhibit advanced liver fibrosis through a variety of modulations, such as targeting specific chemokines [58], cytokines [59], and even immune CD8⁺ T cells [60]. However, both pathogenic and suppression properties of intrahepatic CD8⁺ T cells have been highlighted in liver fibrosis/cirrhosis progression [61], and the functional and phenotypical characteristics of the CD8⁺ T cells associated with positive benefit in the liver disease are largely unknown. Albillos et al. [20] used murine diet-induced nonalcoholic steatohepatitis model (NASH) [2], a currently the leading cause of chronic liver disease worldwide [62], and mainly characterized lobular inflammation and hepatocyte ballooning [63], demonstrating a direct role of CD8⁺ T cells in fibrosis resolution by promoting HSC apoptosis in a CCR5-dependent manner [63], primarily highlighting the undefined role of liver-resident CD8⁺ T cells in the fibrotic/cirrhotic liver niche.

Also, in a recent preliminary study, tracking CD8⁺ T cells with immunofluorescence staining in the DEN mouse model to examine the dynamic changes of intrahepatic CD8⁺ T cells during the model disease development, we curiously found that CD8⁺ T cells were relatively higher in the fibrotic phase (3–5 weeks post-DEN) compared to their in the cirrhotic phase (3–5 weeks post-DEN) where dropping after 7 weeks post-DEN (**Figure 3A** and **Ba, b**), supporting that hepatic resident CD8⁺ T cells may have beneficial role for liver fibrosis/cirrhosis [20], maybe hinting a previously unappreciated role of hepatic resident CD8⁺ T cells in promoting injured liver tissue repair, need to be further investigated.

5. Concluding remarks

This chapter collectively delivers information about the DEN-induced liver fibrosis/cirrhosis in a small amount (0.014%) of water drinking diet chemical (DEN)-induced hepatic fibrosis, cirrhosis and carcinogenesis mouse model and clinical implications, and provides additional insights into the liver possibility of the positive effect of CD8⁺ T cells in the animal model-associated pathogenesis. The sequence of pathophysiological alterations in the model has a high similarity to what happens in humans. In comparison to other mouse models, the DEN-induced liver fibrosis-cirrhosis-HCC model on a natural genetic background C57BL/6 inbred mice sounds favorable, and prolonged application of DEN to induce hepatic inflammatory response and immune CD8⁺ T cell activation after a period of latency are beneficial for endogenous HSP cells (NG2⁺ HSP) mobilization and survival. Based on our experience and on a multitude of independent studies in the field, we recommend that for treatment strategies not inhibit but regulate inflammation and immune CD8⁺ T-cells during liver fibrosis/cirrhosis development. Alternatively, the use of male mice at middle age (approximately 8–10 weeks old) and body weight of the animals should be regularly measured and documented (approximately 22–25 g), and the extent of pathological features (evolution from homeostasis to fibrosis to cirrhosis to HCC formation) should always be histologically proven and documented. Further studies are warranted to identify the specific signaling or molecules that contribute to the development of hepatic homeostasis to fibrosis, then cirrhosis and finally cancer (HCC) in the liver.

Acknowledgements

This work was supported by grants from the National Natural Science Foundation of China (81873586) and the Army Medical University of China (2021-20180-52).

Conflict of interest

The authors declare no conflicts of interest.

Abbreviations

ACLF	acute-on-chronic liver failure
ALD	alcohol-associated liver disease
CDC	Centers for Disease Control
DEN	diethylnitrosamine
DILI	drug-induced liver injury
DLC	decompensated liver cirrhosis

ESLD	end-stage liver disease
HBV	hepatitis B virus
HCC	hepatocyte cellular carcinoma
H&E	hematoxylin-eosin
HSCs	hepatic stellate cells
NAFLD	nonalcoholic fatty liver disease
NG2-HSPs	neuroglia antigen 2-expressing hepatic stem/progenitor cells
TUNEL	terminal deoxynucleotidyl transferase (TdT) dUTP Nick-End Labeling

Author details

Min Yan[1,2], Deyu Hu[1,3], Zhenyu Wu[1], Jiejuan Lai[1], Leida Zhang[1], Hongyu Zhang[1], Sijin Li[2*] and Lianhua Bai[1,2,3*]

1 Hepatobiliary Institute, Southwest Hospital, Army Medical University, Chongqing, China

2 Department of Nuclear Medicine, The First Hospital of Shanxi Medical University, Taiyuan, China

3 Bioengineering College, Chongqing University, Chongqing, China

*Address all correspondence to: lisjnm123@163.com and qqg63@outlook.com

References

[1] Byrnes K, Blessinger S, Bailey NT. Therapeutic regulation of autophagy in hepatic metabolism. Acta Pharmaceutica Sinica B. 2022;**12**:33-49. DOI: 10.1016/j.apsb.2021.07.021

[2] Faccioli LAP, Dias ML, Paranhos BA. Liver cirrhosis: An overview of experimental models in rodents. Life Sciences. 2022;**301**:120615. DOI: 10.1016/j.lfs.2022.120615

[3] Habash NW, Sehrawat TS, Shah VH. Epigenetics of alcohol-related liver diseases. JHEP Report. 2022;**4**(5):100466. DOI: 10.1016/j.jhepr.2022.100466

[4] Khanam A, Tang LSY, Kottilil S. Programmed death 1 expressing $CD8^+$ $CXCR5^+$ follicular T cells constitute effector rather than exhaustive phenotype in patients with chronic hepatitis B. Hepatology. 2022;**75**:690-708. DOI: 10.1002/hep.32210

[5] GBD. 2017 cirrhosis collaborators. The global, regional, and national burden of cirrhosis by cause in 195 countries and territories, 1990-2017: A systematic analysis for the Global Burden of Disease Study 2017. Lancet Gastroenterología y Hepatología. 2020;**5**:245-266. DOI: 10.1016/S2468-1253(19)30349-8

[6] Hou X, Li Y, Yuan H. Therapeutic effect and safety of granulocyte colony-stimulating factor therapy for acute-on-chronic liver failure: A systematic review and meta-analysis of randomized controlled trials. Frontiers in Medicine (Lausanne). 2021;**8**:784240. DOI: 10.3389/fmed.2021.784240

[7] Smith A, Baumgartner K, Bositis C. Cirrhosis: Diagnosis and management. American Family Physician. 2019;**100**: 759-770

[8] Seto WK, Lo YR, Pawlotsky JM. Chronic hepatitis B virus infection. Lancet. 2018;**392**:2313-2324. DOI: 10.1016/S0140-6736(18)31865-8

[9] Liu J, Zhang S, Wang Q. Seroepidemiology of hepatitis B virus infection in 2 million men aged 21-49 years in rural China: A population-based, cross-sectional study. The Lancet Infectious Diseases. 2016;**16**:80-86. DOI: 10.1016/S1473-3099(15)00218-2

[10] Huang F, Ma W, Zheng H. Early risk factors for extrapulmonary organ injury in adult COVID-19 patients. Annals of Translational Medicine. 2021;**9**:701. DOI: 10.21037/atm-21-1561

[11] Kamm DR, McCommis KS. Hepatic stellate cells in physiology and pathology. The Journal of Physiology. 2022;**600**:1825-1837. DOI: 10.1113/JP281061

[12] Newsome PN, Fox R, King AL. Granulocyte colony-stimulating factor and autologous CD133-positive stem-cell therapy in liver cirrhosis (REALISTIC): An open-label, randomised, controlled phase 2 trial. The Lancet Gastroenterology & Hepatology. 2018;**3**:25-36. DOI: 10.1016/S2468-1253(17)30326-6

[13] Zhao L, Chen S, Shi X. A pooled analysis of mesenchymal stem cell-based therapy for liver disease. Stem Cell Research & Therapy. 2018;**91**:72. DOI: 10.1186/s13287-018-0816-2

[14] Zhang Y, Li Y, Li Z. Mesenchymal stem cells: Potential application for the treatment of hepatic cirrhosis. Stem Cell Research & Therapy. 2018;**91**:59. DOI: 10.1186/s13287-018-0814-4

[15] Lanthier N. Haemopoietic stem cell therapy in cirrhosis: The end of the story? The Lancet Gastroenterology & Hepatology. 2018;**3**:3-5. DOI: 10.1016/S2468-1253(17)30359-X

[16] Terai S, Tsuchiya A. Status of and candidates for cell therapy in liver cirrhosis: Overcoming the "point of no return" in advanced liver cirrhosis. Journal of Gastroenterology. 2017;**52**:129-140. DOI: 10.1007/s00535-016-1258-1

[17] Zhang L, Zhou D, Li J. Effects of bone marrow-derived mesenchymal stem cells on hypoxia and the transforming growth factor beta 1 (TGFβ-1) and SMADs pathway in a mouse model of cirrhosis. Medical Science Monitor. 2019;**25**:7182-7190. DOI: 10.12659/MSM.916428

[18] Chen Q, You X, Yang W. Survival of endogenous hepatic stem/progenitor cells in liver tissues during liver cirrhosis. Life Sciences. 2020;**241**:117121. DOI: 10.1016/j.lfs.2019.117121

[19] Tan J, You Y, Linli Z. Water diet DEN-induced liver fibrosis-cirrhosis-cancer mouse model. Journal of Modern Medicine and Health. 2015;**31**:812-813

[20] Albillos A, Martin-Mateos R, Merwe SV. Cirrhosis-associated immune dysfunction. Nature Reviews. Gastroenterology & Hepatology. 2022;**19**(2):112-134. DOI: 10.1038/s41575-021-00520-7

[21] Uehara T, Pogribny IP, Rusyn I. The DEN and CCl4-induced mouse model of fibrosis and inflammation-associated hepatocellular carcinoma. Current Protocols in Pharmacology. 2014;**66**:14.30.1-14.30.10. DOI: 10.1002/0471141755.ph1430s66

[22] Mohamad MI, Desoky IA, Ahmed Zaki K. Pterostilbene ameliorates the disrupted Adars expression and improves liver fibrosis in DEN-induced liver injury in Wistar rats: A novel potential effect [published correction appears in Gene. 2022 Mar 1;813:146145]. Gene. 2022;**813**:146124. DOI: 10.1016/j.gene.2021.146124

[23] Filali-Mouncef Y, Hunter C, Roccio F. The ménage à trois of autophagy, lipid droplets and liver disease. Autophagy. 2022;**18**(1):50-72. DOI: 10.1080/15548627.2021.1895658

[24] Peto R, Gray R, Brantom P. Effects on 4080 rats of chronic ingestion of N-nitrosodiethylamine or N-nitrosodimethylamine: A detailed dose-response study. Cancer Research. 1991;**51**:6415-6451

[25] Williams GM, Iatropoulos MJ, Jeffrey AM. Mechanistic basis for nonlinearities and thresholds in rat liver carcinogenesis by the DNA-reactive carcinogens 2-acetylaminofluorene and diethylnitrosamine. Toxicologic Pathology. 2000;**28**:388-395. DOI: 10.1177/019262330002800306

[26] Magee PN. Toxic liver injury; inhibition of protein synthesis in rat liver by dimethylnitrosamine in vivo. The Biochemical Journal. 1958;**70**:606-611. DOI: 10.1042/bj0700606

[27] George J, Rao KR, Stern R. Dimethylnitrosamine-induced liver injury in rats: The early deposition of collagen. Toxicology. 2001;**156**:129-138. DOI: 10.1016/s0300-483x(00)00352-8

[28] Melhem MF, Kazanecki ME, Rao KN. Genetics and diet: Synergism in hepatocarcinogenesis in rats. Journal of the American College of Nutrition. 1990;**9**:168-173. DOI: 10.1080/07315724.1990.10720367

[29] Wilkins RW. New drug therapies in arterial hypertension. Annals of Internal

Medicine. 1952;**37**(6):1144-1155. DOI: 10.7326/0003-4819-37-6-1144

[30] Barnes JM, Magee PN. Some toxic properties of dimethylnitrosamine. British Journal of Industrial Medicine. 1954;**11**:167-174. DOI: 10.1136/oem.11.3.167

[31] Magee PN, Barnes JM. The production of malignant primary hepatic tumours in the rat by feeding dimethylnitrosamine. British Journal of Cancer. 1956;**10**:114-122. DOI: 10.1038/bjc.1956.15

[32] Druckrey H, Preussmann R, Ivankovic S. Organotrope carcinogene Wirkungen bei 65 verschiedenen N-Nitroso-Verbindungen an BD-Ratten [Organotropic carcinogenic effects of 65 various N-nitroso-compounds on BD rats]. Zeitschrift für Krebsforschung. 1967;**69**:103-201

[33] Arlt JJ, Bongs K, Sengstock K. Bose-Einstein condensation in dilute atomic gases. Die Naturwissenschaften. 2002;**89**:47-56. DOI: 10.1007/s00114-001-0277-8

[34] Kizer DE. Precancerous changes in the activity of enzymes associated with tryptophan metabolism and their relevancy to hepatocarcinogenesis. Annals of the New York Academy of Sciences. 1963;**103**:1127-1136. DOI: 10.1111/j.1749-6632.1963.tb53763.x

[35] Zhang H, Siegel CT, Shuai L. Repair of liver mediated by adult mouse liver neuro-glia antigen 2-positive progenitor cell transplantation in a mouse model of cirrhosis. Scientific Reports. 2016;**6**:21783. DOI: 10.1038/srep21783

[36] Foerster F, Gairing SJ, Müller L. NAFLD-driven HCC: Safety and efficacy of current and emerging treatment options. Journal of Hepatology. 2022;**76**:446-457. DOI: 10.1016/j.jhep.2021.09.007

[37] de Carvalho Ribeiro M, Szabo G. Role of the inflammasome in liver disease. Annual Review of Pathology. 2022;**17**:345-365. DOI: 10.1146/annurev-pathmechdis-032521-102529

[38] Li D, Xie J, Hong D. Efficacy and safety of ligation-assisted endoscopic submucosal resection combined with endoscopic ultrasonography for treatment of rectal neuroendocrine tumors. Scandinavian Journal of Gastroenterology. Feb 2, 2022 [Epub]. DOI: 10.1080/00365521.2022.2033828

[39] Rappaport AM, MacPhee PJ, Fisher MM. The scarring of the liver acini (Cirrhosis). Tridimensional and microcirculatory considerations. Virchows Archive. A, Pathological Anatomy and Histopathology. 1983;**402**:107-137. DOI: 10.1007/BF00695054

[40] Prokudina ES, Maslov LN, Naryzhnaya NV. Prospects of application of remote preconditioning at heart revascularization. Kardiologiia. 2017;**57**:57-61

[41] Carvalho JR, Verdelho Machado M. New insights about albumin and liver disease. Annals of Hepatology. 2018;**17**:547-560. DOI: 10.5604/01.3001.0012.0916

[42] Tsochatzis EA, Bosch J, Burroughs AK. Liver cirrhosis. Lancet. 2014;**383**:1749-1761. DOI: 10.1016/S0140-6736(14)60121-5

[43] Lee DY, Yun SM, Song MY. Administration of steamed and freeze-dried mature silkworm larval powder prevents hepatic fibrosis and hepatocellular carcinogenesis by blocking TGF-β/STAT3 signaling cascades in rats. Cell. 2020;**9**:568. DOI: 10.3390/cells9030568

[44] Chen Q, You Y, Zhang Y. Hepatocyte growth factor mediates a novel form of hepatic stem/progenitor cell-induced tolerance in a rat xenogeneic liver rejection model. International Immunopharmacology. 2021;**90**:107180. DOI: 10.1016/j.intimp.2020.107180

[45] Iwakiri Y. Pathophysiology of portal hypertension. Clinics in Liver Disease. 2014;**18**:281-291. DOI: 10.1016/j.cld.2013.12.001

[46] Khanna R, Sarin SK. Non-cirrhotic portal hypertension—Diagnosis and management. Journal of Hepatology. 2014;**60**:421-441. DOI: 10.1016/j.jhep.2013.08.013

[47] Iannacone M, Guidotti LG. Immunobiology and pathogenesis of hepatitis B virus infection. Nature Reviews. Immunology. 2022;**22**:19-32. DOI: 10.1038/s41577-021-00549-4

[48] Juneja P, Tripathi DM, Kaur S. Revisiting the gut-liver axis: Gut lymphatic system in liver cirrhosis and portal hypertension. American Journal of Physiology. Gastrointestinal and Liver Physiology. 2022;**322**:G473-G479. DOI: 10.1152/ajpgi.00271.2021

[49] Bonnel AR, Bunchorntavakul C, Reddy KR. Immune dysfunction and infections in patients with cirrhosis. Clinical Gastroenterology and Hepatology. 2011;**9**:727-738. DOI: 10.1016/j.cgh.2011.02.031

[50] Albillos A, Lario M, Álvarez-Mon M. Cirrhosis-associated immune dysfunction: Distinctive features and clinical relevance. Journal of Hepatology. 2014;**61**:1385-1396. DOI: 10.1016/j.jhep.2014.08.010

[51] Kumar R, Krishnamoorthy TL, Tan HK. Change in model for end-stage liver disease score at two weeks, as an indicator of mortality or liver transplantation at 60 days in acute-on-chronic liver failure. Gastroenterology Report (Oxf). 2015;**3**:122-127. DOI: 110.1093/gastro/gou075

[52] Lahmer T, Peçanha-Pietrobom PM, Schmid RM. Invasive fungal infections in acute and chronic liver impairment: A systematic review. Mycoses. 2022;**65**:140-151. DOI: 10.1111/myc.13403

[53] Martin-Mateos R, Alvarez-Mon M, Albillos A. Dysfunctional immune response in acute-on-chronic liver failure: It takes two to tango. Frontiers in Immunology. 2019;**10**:973. DOI: 10.3389/fimmu.2019.00973

[54] Orci LA, Sanduzzi-Zamparelli M, Caballol B. Incidence of hepatocellular carcinoma in patients with nonalcoholic fatty liver disease: A systematic review, meta-analysis, and meta-regression. Clinical Gastroenterology and Hepatology. 2022;**20**:283-292.e10. DOI: 10.1016/j.cgh.2021.05.002

[55] Huang X, Wang H, Zhang W. Verification of hepatitis B-related hepatocellular carcinoma predictive models to evaluate the risk of HCC in patients with liver cirrhosis under antiviral treatment. European Journal of Gastroenterology & Hepatology. 2022;**34**:546-552. DOI: 10.1097/MEG.0000000000002302

[56] Ko FY, Tsai SJ, Yang AC. Association of CD8 T cells with depression and anxiety in patients with liver cirrhosis. International Journal of Psychiatry in Medicine. 2013;**45**:15-29. DOI: 10.2190/PM.45.1.b

[57] Arthur MJ. Reversibility of liver fibrosis and cirrhosis following treatment for hepatitis C. Gastroenterology. 2002;**122**:1525-1528. DOI: 10.1053/gast.2002.33367

[58] Tacke F, Weiskirchen R. An update on the recent advances in antifibrotic therapy. Expert Review of Gastroenterology & Hepatology. 2018;**12**:1143-1152. DOI: 10.1080/17474124.2018.1530110

[59] Dewidar B, Meyer C, Dooley S. TGF-β in hepatic stellate cell activation and liver fibrogenesis-updated 2019. Cell. 2019;**8**:1419. DOI: 10.3390/cells8111419

[60] Breuer DA, Pacheco MC, Washington MK. $CD8^+$ T cells regulate liver injury in obesity-related nonalcoholic fatty liver disease. American Journal of Physiology. Gastrointestinal and Liver Physiology. 2020;**318**:G211-G224. DOI: 10.1152/ajpgi.00040.2019

[61] Kefalakes H, Horgan XJ, Jung MK. Liver-resident bystander $CD8^+$ T cells contribute to liver disease pathogenesis in chronic hepatitis D virus infection. Gastroenterology. 2021;**161**:1567-1583.e9. DOI: 10.1053/j.gastro.2021.07.027

[62] Anstee QM, Reeves HL, Kotsiliti E. From NASH to HCC: Current concepts and future challenges. Nature Reviews. Gastroenterology & Hepatology. 2019;**16**:411-428. DOI: 10.1038/s41575-019-0145-7

[63] Alexopoulos AS, Crowley MJ, Wang Y. Glycemic control predicts severity of hepatocyte ballooning and hepatic fibrosis in nonalcoholic fatty liver disease. Hepatology. 2021;**74**:1220-1233. DOI: 10.1002/hep.31806

Chapter 5

Intervention of PAR-2 Mediated CGRP in Animal Model of Visceral Hyperalgesia

Manoj Shah

Abstract

Protease-activated receptor-2 (PAR-2) mediates calcitonin gene-related peptide (CGRP) release and collectively plays a crucial role in inflammation-induced visceral hyperalgesia (VH). The present review chapter outlines the substantial advances that elucidated the underlying role of PAR-2 and CGRP in gut inflammation-induced VH and highlights their relevancies in the management of VH. PAR-2 is expressed in a wide range of gastrointestinal cells and its activation on primary afferent nerves by tryptase, trypsin or cathepsin-S is the key mechanism of sensitization during intestinal inflammation. The activated PAR-2 sensitizes transient receptor potential vanilloid subtype-1 receptors and triggers the release of substance-P (SP) and CGRP that are involved both in the transmission and modulation of VH. Approximately, two-thirds of sensory neurons express PAR-2 and 40% of the PAR-2-expressing sensory neurons also express SP and CGRP. Accumulating set of experiments devised that the blockade or antagonism of PAR-2 in inflammatory diseases of the gut depicts double advantages of reducing inflammation and VH. Simultaneously, the uses of CGRP-antagonists inhibit VH and completely suppress PAR-2-agonists-induced intestinal inflammation in animals. However, further study is imperative to improve our understanding of the blockade or antagonism of PAR-2 and CGRP release before its implication as a novel therapeutic for the clinical management of VH in human patients.

Keywords: PAR-2, CGRP, intestinal inflammation, visceral hyperalgesia, activation

1. Introduction

Visceral hyperalgesia (VH) is a pathological state of inflammatory bowel diseases (IBDs) and irritable bowel syndrome (IBS) or other functional bowel disorders, in which sensory threshold for abdominal pain and discomfort decreases due to tissue injury, inflammation, and persistent exposure of tissues/organ to noxious stimuli. In this state, the continuous release of inflammatory mediators results in sensitization of primary afferents and abdominal pain, both during the acute flare of diseases and their remission [1, 2]. Despite several proposed factors including inflammation, psychology and aberrant sensory-motor function of the gut contribute to peripheral and central sensitization [3], the exact underlying mechanism of VH has not been fully elucidated. The cell-membrane protease-activated receptor-2 (PAR-2) mediates calcitonin gene-related peptide (CGRP) release, and their associated roles in neurogenic inflammation-induced sensitization could be of great interest for the researchers to address this persistent nature of VH.

A G-protein coupled receptor PAR-2, distributed throughout the gastrointestinal (GI) tract, is activated particularly by proteases such as tryptase, trypsin, and cathepsin-S [4–6]. PAR-2 activation on several cells (epithelial cells, endothelial cells, neutrophils, macrophages, monocytes, mast cells, fibroblasts, neurons, dendritic cells, lymphocytes, etc.) could lead to the release of cytokines, chemokines, prostaglandins [7], as well as CGRP and substance-P (SP) in the enteric neurons and afferent neurons [8, 9]. Numerous reports indicated the diverse SP and CGRP expressions within the dorsal root ganglia (DRG) and spinal neurons during colitis and ileitis [10–15]. The expressions of SP and CGRP within the gut not only excite extrinsic afferents but also perpetuate the central transmission of nociceptive traffic between afferent neurons and higher-order neurons in the spinal cord and brainstem [16]. Thus, it is worthwhile to consider the key role of PAR-2 in the release of CGRP, which subsequently triggers neurogenic inflammation mediated VH.

Currently, the pharmacotherapy for VH is unsatisfactory because of its unknown precise mechanism. Earlier study suggests that the blockade of PAR-2at the periphery and/or the inhibition of luminal protease activity may be of interest for treating the VH [17]. Likewise, the administration of CGRP antagonists inhibits VH in animals [18, 19]. Therefore, the blockade or antagonism of either PAR-2 or CGRP may be a promising therapeutic target for VH. This review chapter explores the important roles of PAR-2 and PAR-2-mediated CGRP during inflammatory gut and their antagonism or blockade for the treatment of VH.

2. PAR-2 activation in the gastrointestinal tract

PAR-2 is activated through proteolytic cleavage by specific serine proteases, such as trypsin and mast cell (MC)-tryptase [4] and lysosomal macrophagic cysteine protease cathepsin-S [5, 6]. PAR-2 is generally expressed in the basolateral and apical side of epithelial cells [20], fibroblasts, MCs, smooth muscle cells, endothelial cells of the GI tract [21], enteric sensory neurons, terminals of mesenteric afferent nerves, and immune cells [17]. The higher number of mast cells and mast cell tryptase in biopsied colonic tissues enhanced the PAR-2 activity to regulate CGRP, SP, and VIP expressions resulting in symptoms associated with IBD [22]. Recently, Hassler et al. [23] suggested that PAR2-expressed sensory neurons are a key target for mechanical and spontaneous pain triggered by the release of endogenous proteases from the many immune cells. In-vitro study exhibits the up-regulation of PAR-2 expression in cultured endothelial cells of human umbilical vein treated with TNF-α, IL-1α, and bacterial lipopolysaccharide in a dose-dependent manner [24]. Therefore, it is important to note that PAR-2 activation on intestinal immunocytes induces acute enteritis [9, 25] while its neuronal expression incites neurogenic inflammation [26, 27].

2.1 Role of PAR-2 in inflammation

PAR-2 seems essential in the interplay between nerves, immunocytes, MCs, and epithelial cells within the luminal wall during GI diseases [17]. Histopathologically, PAR-2-agonists (SLIGRL) induced acute colitis has been observed with erythema, granulocyte infiltrations and thickened colonic wall [25, 28], the colonic tissue sampled from the PAR-2 knockout mice that are infused intracolonically with 2,4,6-trinitrobenzene sulfonic acid (TNBS) showed lower myeloperoxidase activities, microscopic- and macroscopic-damage scores [29]. Mediators such as intracellular- and vascular cell adhesion-molecule-1 were decreased while cyclooxygenase-1 was increased in the PAR-2 knockout mice, which clearly confirms the pro-inflammatory role of PAR-2. Notably, PAR-2, inactive during colitis, has been expressed for inducing VH after resolution of colitis [30]. Furthermore, PAR-2 has also been over-expressed in biopsies obtained from ulcerative colitis (UC) and CD patients, which strongly suggests its intricate role in IBDs [31–33].

2.2 Effects of PAR-2 on gastrointestinal functions

PAR-2 modulates GI functions, such as motility, ionic exchange, paracellular permeability, sensory functions, and inflammation [34]. The excitatory, as well as inhibitory actions of PAR-2-agonists on isolated smooth muscles, have been devised earlier [35, 36]. In-vitro, PAR-2 activation shows a region-specific role because it enhances the contractibility of gastric smooth muscles and reduces the contractility of circular and longitudinal colonic smooth muscles in mice [35, 37]. However, the intraperitoneal administration of PAR-2-agonists accelerated GI transit in mice [38]. Moreover, Mall et al. (2002) reported that PAR-2 activation on the enterocytes triggers intestinal water secretion through a direct cellular mechanism, while Kong et al. [20] described the same by a prostaglandin E2-dependent mechanism. Additionally, activated PAR-2 stimulates mucus secretion by a nerve-mediated mechanism [39]. It weakens the intestinal barrier, resulting in an increased passage of fluids or even microorganisms across the gut mucosa. The intracolonic administration of PAR-2-agonist in mice increases colonic permeability and results in a general inflammatory response [25, 34].

3. CGRP-receptors and their distribution

CGRP-receptor is a heterotrimeric complex, composed of calcitonin receptor-like receptor (CLR), receptor activity-modifying protein-1, and a small intracellular protein component and receptor component protein. CLR, a classical G-protein linked receptor, couples through adenylyl cyclase [40]. CGRP is expressed throughout the peripheral and central nervous systems (CNS). Of the two forms, α-CGRP is mainly expressed in the CNS, especially in striatum, amygdalae, hypothalamus, colliculi, brainstem, cerebellum, and trigeminal complex [41–43], while β-CGRP is primarily expressed in the enteric neurons and vascular smooth muscle cells [44, 45]. Interestingly, α-CGRP is also found to be expressed in primary spinal afferent C- and Aδ-fibers [46].

The majority of spinal afferents innervated into the GI tract express CGRP and SP [47]. CGRP has been reported to be expressed markedly higher in the lumbosacral DRG and spinal cord dorsal horn (SCDH) during visceral inflammation [11, 48]. Zhang et al. [49] confirmed the absence of secondary hyperalgesia in the mice missing α-CGRP expression in the CNS. The SP and CGRP released from afferent terminals lead to neurogenic inflammation at the peripheral sites, resulting in MCs degranulation, plasma extravasation, and arteriolar vasodilation [50]. CGRP causes vasodilatation via its receptors on the smooth muscle cells at peripheral synapses. However, at central synapses, it acts postsynaptically on the second-order neurons to transmit pain via the brainstem and midbrain to higher cortical pain regions [51].

3.1 CGRP modulates mast cell functions

CGRP is secreted from non-myelinated C-fibers and thinly myelinated Aδ-fibers originating from DRG neurons [52]. Sun et al. [53] showed peak CGRP levels in the colonic tissues, spinal cord, and hypothalamus of rats with IBS, and its correlation with VH. Our earlier studies also demonstrated the remarkably higher CGRP expression in DRG and spinal cord that was correlated with VH in the TNBS-induced ileitis rats and goats, respectively [13, 15]. Therefore, CGRP and CGRP-receptors are found to be involved in the transmission and modulation of pain in the periphery and CNS [54, 55].

MCs that reside near the nerve fibers are true candidates for modulating neural activity and nociception [56]. The mediators such as SP, CGRP, vasoactive intestinal protein (VIP), dopamine, and arachidonic acid are able to influence MCs activation. The aforementioned mediators act on nociceptors, send signals to the CNS, and cause the simultaneous central release of SP and CGRP [57], which further activate MCs, and create a bidirectional positive feedback-loop for resultant neurogenic inflammation [58].

3.2 CGRP-release mediated by PAR-2

Activated PAR-2 sensitizes Transient Receptor Potential Vanilloid subtype-1 receptors (TRPV-1) and triggers the release of sensory CGRP and SP [59]. CGRP and SP released from intestinal afferent terminals cause vascular dilatation, plasma extravasation, granulocyte infiltrations, and neurogenic inflammation [8, 9, 60]. An earlier study [8] reported that PAR-2-agonists-induced edema was entirely mediated by the release of SP and CGRP from sensory neurons and further activation of neurokinin-1 (NK-1)- and CGRP-receptors on endothelial cells. In DRG, PAR-2 co-expresses with TRPV-1, TRPV-4, TRPA-1 (Transient Receptor Potential Cation Channel, Subfamily-A, Member-1), SP and CGRP [8, 61, 62]. It is also reported that 63% of sensory neurons express PAR-2 and up to 40% of them express both SP and CGRP [8]. Activated PAR-2 transmits C-fiber afferent input to the SCDH for the release of excitatory amino acids and neuropeptides from the central terminals [63].

3.3 Role of CGRP in sensitization

Afferent fibers innervating the gut vessels have cell bodies in the DRG. These fibers are peptidergic, containing both CGRP and SP, and have collaterals in enteric ganglia, mucosa, muscularis externa, and sympathetic prevertebral ganglia [64]. SP, CGRP, VIP, and somatostatin act as mediators of neurogenic inflammation in IBDs [65–67]. After stimulation, TRPV-1 depolarizes sensory neurons either directly or indirectly to initiate the release of these neuropeptides from the afferent terminals [68]. TRPV-1-positive nerve fibers co-express with SP, NK-1, and CGRP in mucosa, submucosal layer, deep muscular plexus, circular muscle, myenteric plexus, and longitudinal muscle layer in the rectum and colon of mice [69]. CGRP which is expressed largely in splanchnic afferents and CGRP-immunoreactivities from the GI tract disappears with capsaicin treatment [70]. Interestingly, about 50% of CGRP-immunoreactive extrinsic afferent neurons express SP- or NK-1-immunoreactivities [71] and their expressions fluctuate during colitis [72]. The earlier decrease of the above neuropeptides may be due to their depletion from the peripheral nerve terminals or the damaged nerves at the initial inflammatory stage. CGRP and SP increase during inflammation or afferent nerve stimulation. TNBS-induced colitis/ileitis and or colorectal distension (CRD) results in higher expression of neural activation markers (such as c-Fos, pERK) as well as releases of SP and CGRP in the SCDH that are commonly linked with pain signaling [15, 73, 74].

Plourde et al. [75] confirmed the role of CGRP in pain modulation because intravenously administered CGRP-1-receptor-antagonists (h-CGRP8-37) reversed the sensitization provoked by infusion of intracolonic acetic acid. SP and CGRP may either increase the peripheral sensory gain of extrinsic afferents within the gut or contribute to primary afferent transmission within the CNS [16, 76]. Despite irritation, immune challenge and inflammation cause the release of CGRP and SP from extrinsic afferents and intrinsic neurons within the gut [45, 77], the precise site at which CGRP-receptor and NK-1 mediate visceral pain is not known.

4. Role of PAR-2 in VH

PAR-2 activation in GI resident cells such as MCs, macrophages, or neutrophils induces the release of tiny amounts of inflammatory mediators that sensitizes primary afferents. It regulates vascular tone and causes immense pro- or anti-inflammatory as well as pro-nociceptive effects in somatic or visceral pain [78]. PAR-2 expressed at the peripheral afferent neurons is more importantly involved in inflammation-induced VH [29, 30]. The glial cells of the enteric nervous system play pivotal roles in neuroimmune interactions and modulate enteric neurotransmission, inflammation, and intestinal barrier functions as they express receptors for purines and contain precursors for neurotransmitters such as GABA and NO. They can produce cytokines (TNF-α, IL-1β, IL-6), NGF, and neuropeptides (NK-1, SP, CGRP) after their activation. Both PAR-2 and proinflammatory cytokines impair the epithelial barrier by decreasing tight junction protein expression and consequently facilitate the entry of luminal aggressors perpetuating inflammation and pain [9].

PAR-2 expressed in enterocytes increases permeability, which is linked with the immune activation and generation of VH [25, 79]. It is found that PAR-2-agonists evoke the transient depolarization of submucosal enteric neurons with long-lasting hyperexcitability in guinea pigs [80]. Similarly, intracolonically administered PAR-2 agonist (SLIGRL-NH2, 100 μg/mouse) increased intestinal permeability and VH in mice [81]. The intracolonic administration of sub-inflammatory doses of PAR-2-agonist led to prolonging the VH in response to CRD in rats [78]. PAR-2 activation on enteric neurons is also directly responsible for the development of VH as it conveys nociceptive signals for the excitability of submucosal neurons, colonic projections of DRG, and jejunal afferent neurons [7]. Shi et al. [82] reported PAR-2 activation and higher CGRP levels in the serum and colonic tissue during VH in a rat model of IBS. Accumulating set of evidence suggests that protease activity is remarkably prominent in diarrheic-IBS and UC patients. The fecal supernatant or colonic biopsies from these patients when infused intracolonally into rodents resulted in higher intestinal permeability, mucosal inflammation, and subsequent VH through a PAR-2 activation mechanism [83–86], while the same treatment failed to cause the VH in the PAR-2 knockout mice [83]. **Table 1** summarizes the findings of preclinical studies that intervened in the effects of PAR-2 on underlying VH.

PAR	Agonist/ antagonist	Species (hypersensitivity model)	Study type	Effects	Ref.
PAR-2	Agonist (SLIGRL-NH2)	Mice (PAR2-agonist)	In vivo	↑ hyperalgesia	[39]
PAR-2	Agonist (SLIGRL-NH2, Tc-NH2, trypsin, tryptase)	Mice, rat (PAR-2-agonist)	KO	↑ hyperalgesia, absent in KO mice	[87]
PAR-2	Agonist (SLIGRL-NH2, trypsin)	Rat (PAR2-agonist)	In-vivo	↑ hyperalgesia	[78]
PAR-2	PAR-2 agonists (trypsin, tryptase, and a selective PAR-2-activating peptide)	Mice received intracolonically PAR-2 agonists	KO	Colonic administration of PAR-2 agonists up-regulated PAR-2 expression and induced colonic inflammatory reaction and permeability.	[25]
PAR-2	Agonist (SLIGR)	Intracolonic infusion to mice	In-vivo	Colonic inflammation and enhanced colonic permeability, while the intravenous injection of CGRP antagonist, i.e., CGRP (8–37) prevented PAR-2 induced colonic inflammation.	[9]
PAR-2	Agonist (SL-NH2, trypsin, tryptase)	Guinea pig submucosal neurons (PAR-2-agonist)	Ex-vivo	↑ neuron excitability	[80]
PAR-2	Agonist (SLIGR)	Intracolonic infusion of SLIGR (5 and 100 μg per mouse)	In-vivo	At lower dose, SLIGRL increased colonic permeability while higher dose resulted in colonic inflammation	[79]
PAR-2	Agonist (2-furoyl-LIGRL-NH2)	Mice (capsaicin)	KO	↑ hyperalgesia, absent in KO	[88]
PAR-2	Antagonist (ENMD-1068)	Mice (IBS-supernatant)	KO	↓ hypersensitivity, absent in KO	[83]

PAR	Agonist/ antagonist	Species (hypersensitivity model)	Study type	Effects	Ref.
PAR-2	PAR-2 deficient	TNBS- and dextran sodium sulfate-induced colitis in mice	KO	Endogenous PAR-2 activation controls leukocyte recruitment in the colon and thus possesses a new potential therapeutic target for the treatment of IBD.	[29]
PAR-2	PAR-2 activation	TNBS-induced colitis rats	In-vivo	PAR-2 activation resulted in colitis and VH	[30]
PAR-2	Mediators from colonic biopsies of diarrhea-predominant IBS patients	Mice DRG (IBS-D supernatant)	KO	↑ neuron excitability, absent in KO mice	[89]
PAR-2	Colono-scopic biopsies	IBS-D and IBS-C patients	In-vivo	Elevated PAR-2 expression to regulate the expression of CGRP, VIP and SP resulting in symptoms associated with IBD	[22]
PAR-2	IntracolonicPAR-2 agonist (SLIGRL-NH2, 100 μg/mouse)	PI-IBS Mouse Model	In-vivo	↑ intestinal permeability and VH	[81]
PAR-2	PAR-2 activation	TNBS-induced post-inflammation irritable bowel syndrome (PI-IBS) rats	In--vivo	↑ visceral hypersensitivity	[90]
PAR-2	PAR-2 activation	TNBS-induced ileitis goat	In-vivo	↑ visceral hypersensitivity	[15]

Abbreviations: DRG, dorsal root ganglia; IBD, inflammatory bowel diseases; IBS, irritable bowel syndrome; KO, Knock-out; PAR-2, Protease-activated receptor-2.

Table 1.
Preclinical studies investigating the effects of protease activated receptor-2 on visceral hyperalgesia.

Currently, the role of cathepsin-S is considered insightful because it activates spinal nociceptive neurons through a PAR-2-dependent mechanism and amplifies VH. Over the years, studies reported that cathepsin-S released from spinal microglial cells during nerve injury or colitis secretes fractalkine, thereby intensifying and maintaining the chronic pain [91, 92].

5. Role of PAR-2 in pain transmission

Proteases directly activate PAR-2 as well as assist other pronociceptive mediators for the subsequent sensitization of afferent fibers [83]. **Figure 1** illustrates the important role of PAR-2 in pain transmission during GI disorders. PAR-2 activation on afferent neurons leads to specific calcium signals that could participate in conveying pain messages [93]. Elmariah et al. [6] reported that cathepsin-S played a role in molecular signaling either alone or together with activated PAR-2. Activation of PAR-2 on DRG by its agonists enhances potassium chloride ions and the capsaicin (TRPV-1 agonist)-evoked release of CGRP [8, 94]. Protease-activated receptor-1 and PAR-2 on enteric afferent fibers facilitate nociceptive input to the CNS, while spinal PAR-2 activation aggravates pain behaviors [21]. These findings strongly suggest that visceral activation of PAR-2 has an important role in sensitizing the second-order neurons at spinal level.

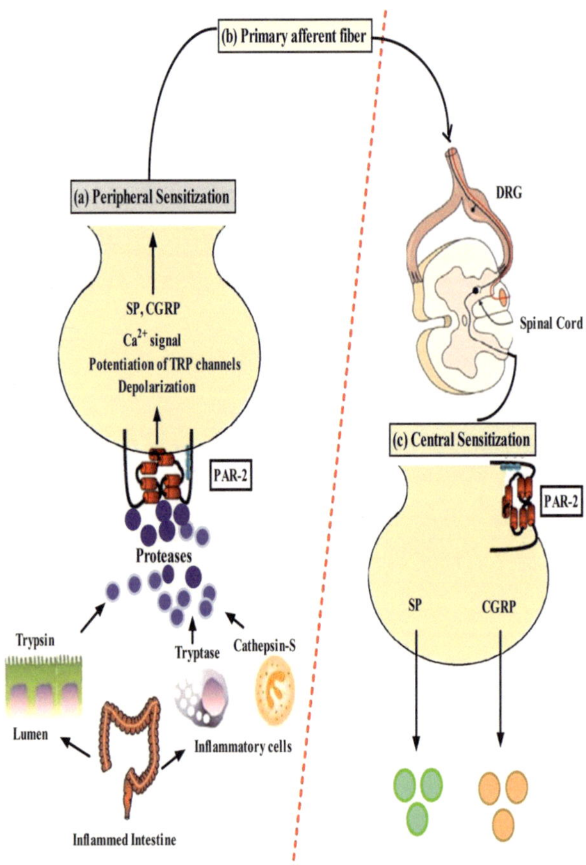

Figure 1.
Role of PAR-2 in pain transmission. (a) Peripheral sensitization. PAR-2 is activated by proteases released from inflammatory and immune cells as well as from mediators of the intestinal lumen. Proteases sensitize neurons to innocuous stimuli. After stimulation, TRPV-1 depolarizes sensory neurons either directly or indirectly to initiate the release of SP and CGRP from the afferent terminals. PAR-2 activation on afferent neurons leads to specific calcium signals. (b) Primary afferent fiber. Pain signal is transmitted along primary afferent fibers to the spinal dorsal horn and subsequently to the brain. (c) Central sensitization. Persistent small-afferent input leads to a central sensitization associated with local release of SP and CGRP. PAR-2, protease-activated receptor-2; TRP, Transient Receptor Potential; Ca^{2+}, calcium ion; SP, substance-P; CGRP, calcitonin gene-related peptide; TRPV-1, Transient Receptor Potential Vanilloid subtype-1.

6. Therapies targeting PAR-2 and CGRP for VH

Researchers have come a long way in terms of understanding and controlling the inflammation-induced VH in experimental animals. An overview of the studies described in the following paragraph is shown in **Table 2**. It is worth mentioning

Targeted substances	Antagonist/ inhibitors	Species (VH model)	Study type	Effects	Ref.
PAR-2	PAR-2 antagonist (GB88)	PAR-2-agonists and TNBS-induced colitis rats	In-vivo	Acute and chronic colitis ↓	[28]
PAR-2	PAR-2 gene deletion	Paw inflammation in Rats and Mice	In-vivo	Hyperalgesia ↓	[87]
PAR-2	PAR-2 agonist (SLIGRL-NH2)	PAR-2 agonist induced colitis and VH	In-vivo	Increased intestinal permeability and the activation of NK_1 receptors.SLIGRL-NH2 induced hyperalgesia was inhibited by a NK_1 receptor antagonist (SR 140333).	[78]
PAR-2	PAR-2 agonist	Intrapancreatic administration of PAR-2	In-vivo	PAR-2 expression in all thoracic DRG. Increased c-FOS expression and pain behaviors.	[95]
PAR-2	PAR-2 antagonist PAR-2 knockout	Colonic biopsy from IBS patients	In-vivo	Supernatants from colonic biopsies of IBS patients showed VH. Serine protease inhibitors and a PAR-2 antagonist inhibited VH. However, VH was absent in PAR-2 knockout mice.	[83]
Protease	Fecal protease	Fecal proteases from IBS-D patients	In-vitro	Increased fecal protease and amylase in patients with IBS-D.	[86]
PAR-2	Serene protease inhibitor and PAR-2 antagonist Knockout	Fecal supernatant from IBS-D patients infused into the colon of mice	In-vivo	Increased VH in mice infused with fecal supernatant while VH was suppressed in mice infused with intracolonic serene protease inhibitor and PAR-2 antagonist.	[96]
PAR-2	PAR-2 antagonist (FSLLRY-NH2, 3 mg/kg daily intraperitoneally for 5 days)	PI-IBS Mouse Model	In-vivo	Intestinal permeability and VH ↓	[81]
CGRP	Intravenous antagonist CGRP [human CGRP-(8–37) Intrathecal administration of hCGRP-(8–37) (mid-lumbar)	Acetic acid induced colitis Intravenous CGRP to induce VH	In-vivo	VH ↓	[18]

Targeted substances	Antagonist/ inhibitors	Species (VH model)	Study type	Effects	Ref.
CGRP	CGRP antagonist (h-CGRP 8–37)	TNBS-induced colitis	In-vivo	VH ↓	[97]
CGRP	Mutant mice lacking α-CGRP or β-CGRP expression	DSS induced colitis	In-vivo	α-CGRP and β-CGRP play a protective role in the generation of spontaneous colitis, supporting a role for both extrinsic and intrinsic CGRP-containing neurons.	[98]
CGRP	CGRP antagonist (hCGRP8–37)	Intraperitoneal acetic acid-induced VH	In-vivo	VH ↓	[99]
CGRP	CGRP antagonist (hCGRP8–37)	TNBS-induced acute colitis rats	In-vivo	Intrathecal administration of hCGRP8–37 reversed the CGRP expressions and alleviated the VH.	[19]
CGRP	EA	Chronic and acute stressed rats with IBS-D	In-vivo	EA attenuates VH in rats with IBS-D through suppressing spinal CGRP.	[53]
CGRP	Shugan decoction (herbal extracts)	A rat model of IBS induced by chronic water avoidance stress	In-vivo	Intragastrically administered Shugan decoction abolished VH by attenuating the PAR-2 and CGRP.	[82]
PAR-2 and CGRP	EA at ST-37 and ST-25	A rat model of IBS induced by chronic water avoidance stress	In-vivo	Attenuation of VH attributed due to decreasing number of MCs and down-regulation of PAR-2, TRPV1, CGRP, SP and Try proteins in the colonic tissues.	[100]
PAR-2 and CGRP	EA at ST-25 and ST-37	TNBS instilled into anus to induce post-inflammation visceral hypersensitivity	In-vivo	EA alleviated visceral hypersensitivity symptoms through downregulation of the PAR-2, SP and CGRP in colonic tissues in post inflammation-IBS rats.	[90]
PAR-2 and CGRP	EA at ST-36	TNBS-induced ileitis	In-vivo	Repetitive EA therapy attenuated visceral hypersensitivity through the suppression of spinal PAR-2 and CGRP in goats.	[15]
CGRP	$F(ab')_2$ fragment antibody (30 mg/kg intraperitoneally)	Chronic Adult Stress in rats Induced by Water Avoidance Stress	In-vivo	A single dose of $F(ab')_2$ fragment antibody inhibited stress-induced colonic hypersensitivity	[101]

Abbreviations: PAR-2, protease-activated receptor-2;TNBS, 2,4,6-trinitrobenzene sulfonic acid; DRG, dorsal root ganglia; NK-1, neurokinin-1;IBS, irritable bowel syndrome; IBS-D, irritable bowel syndrome with diarrhea; CGRP, calcitonin gene-related peptide; α-CGRP, alpha-calcitonin gene-related peptide; β-CGRP, beta-calcitonin gene-related peptide; VH, visceral hyperalgesia; EA, electroacupuncture.

Table 2.
Preclinical studies targeting the antagonism or blockade of PAR-2 and CGRP as a therapeutic strategy for the management of inflammation and visceral hyperalgesia.

that the oral administration of PAR-2-antagonists (GB88) ameliorates acute and chronic colitis induced by PAR-2-agonists and TNBS, respectively, in rats [28]. Several studies have demonstrated that protease inhibitors and PAR-2-antagonists relieve the inflammation and resultant VH in animals [78, 83, 86, 87, 95, 96, 102]. In chronic inflammation and pain syndromes, the blockade of PAR-2 inhibits both pain signals and inflammatory responses [7]. The intraperitoneal administration of PAR-2 antagonist (FSLLRY-NH2, 3 mg/kg daily for 5 days) reversed intestinal permeability and also attenuated VH in PI-IBS mice which confirms the therapeutic potential of PAR-2antagonist in VH [81].

Studies utilizing both CGRP knockout mice and antagonist hCGRP8-37 have confirmed the protective role of CGRP in colitis and devised its insightful roles in hyperalgesia [18, 97, 98, 103]. Intravenously administered hCGRP8-37 attenuated distension-evoked pain responses and completely reversed the sensitization effects in acetic acid-induced acute colitis rats [18]. Julia and Bueno [99] reported that hCGRP8-37 also suppressed the pain in rats provoked by intraperitoneal injection of acetic acid. Furthermore, its intrathecal administration reversed the CGRP expressions and alleviated the VH in both acetic acid-induced acute and TNBS-induced chronic colitis rats [18, 19]. Recently, Noor-Mohammadi et al. [101] reported that the single dose of intraperitoneally administered anti-CGRP, i.e., $F(ab')_2$ fragment antibody attenuated the stress-induced colonic hypersensitivity in rats which confirms the prevailing role of CGRP in persistent visceral pain.

Nowadays, alternative therapies have been attracting attention due to their potential in the treatment of VH. Sun et al. [53] described that electroacupuncture (EA) attenuates VH in rats with diarrheic-IBS by suppressing spinal CGRP. EA therapy also alleviated the VH symptoms through downregulation of the PAR2, SP, and CGRP levels in colon tissues in post-inflammation-IBS rats [90]. Likewise, Deng et al. [100] exhibited that the EA at ST-37 and ST-25 relieved the VH in IBS rats by decreasing the number of MCs and suppressing the expression of PAR-2, TRPV1, CGRP, SP and Try proteins in the colonic tissues. Our recent study also reported the effectiveness of repetitive EA for treating both acute and chronic pain because it down-regulated the PAR-2-mediated CGRP release in the spinal cord [15]. Shi et al. [82] administered Shugan decoction (herbal extracts) intragastrically in rats in IBS model and found that it abolished VH by attenuating the release of PAR-2-mediated CGRP.

7. Conclusions

GI tract is the organ that is exposed frequently to proteases both during physiological and pathophysiological conditions. Besides degradative enzymatic roles, the proteases also act as signaling molecules in various gut diseases. Understanding the exact mechanism of VH is pivotal to identifying the novel efficacious therapy for IBDs. PAR-2 activation by tryptase, trypsin, and cathepsin-S causes the release of CGRP and SP in extrinsic primary afferent fibers and intrinsic enteric neurons [45, 77]. Both CGRP and SP facilitate the excitation of extrinsic afferents as well as participate in the central transmission of nociceptive traffic between afferent neurons and higher-order neurons in the spinal cord and brainstem. The blockade and/or antagonism of PAR-2 and CGRP release can effectively relieve VH in IBDs, IBS, or other functional bowel disorders. Further research is required to deepen our understanding of the blockade or antagonism of PAR-2 or CGRP before these potential therapies can be clinically translated for the management of VH in humans.

Author contributions

The author confirms sole responsibility for the conception, drafting, revision, and the approval of final review chapter.

Conflict of interest

The author declares no conflict of interest.

Abbreviations

CGRP	calcitonin gene-related peptide
CNS	central nervous system
CRD	colorectal distension
DRG	dorsal root ganglia
GI	gastrointestinal
IBD	inflammatory bowel diseases
IBS	irritable bowel syndromes
MC	mast cell
NK-1	neurokinin-1
PAR-2	protease-activated receptor-2
SCDH	spinal cord dorsal horn
SP	substance-P
TNBS	2,4,6-trinitrobenzene sulfonic acid
UC	ulcerative colitis
VH	visceral hyperalgesia
VIP	vasoactive intestinal protein

Author dctails

Manoj Shah
Department of Surgery and Pharmacology, Agriculture and Forestry University, Rampur, Nepal

*Address all correspondence to: mkshah@afu.edu.np

References

[1] Minderhoud IM, Oldenburg B, Wismeijer JA, Van Berge Henegouwen GP, Smout AJPM. IBS-like symptoms in patients with inflammatory bowel disease in remission; relationships with quality of life and coping behavior. Digestive Diseases and Sciences. 2004;**49**(3):469-474

[2] Bielefeldt K, Davis B, Binion DG. Pain and inflammatory bowel disease. Inflammatory Bowel Diseases. 2009;**15**:778-788

[3] Azpiroz F, Bouin M, Camilleri M, Mayer EA, Poitras P, Serra J, et al. Mechanisms of hypersensitivity in IBS and functional disorders. Neurogastroenterology and Motility. 2007;**19**(Suppl. 1):62-88

[4] Ossovskaya VS, Bunnett NW. Protease-activated receptors: Contribution to physiology and disease. Physiological Reviews. 2004;**84**(2):579-621

[5] Reiser J, Adair B, Reinheckel T. Specialized roles for cysteine cathepsins in health and disease. Journal of Clinical Investigation. 2010;**120**:3421-3431

[6] Elmariah SB, Reddy VB, Lerner EA. Cathepsin S signals via PAR2 and generates a novel tethered ligand receptor agonist. PLoS One. 2014;**9**(6):e99702

[7] Vergnolle N. Protease-activated receptors as drug targets in inflammation and pain. Pharmacology & Therapeutics. 2009;**123**(3):292-309

[8] Steinhoff M, Vergnolle N, Young SH, Tognetto M, Amadesi S, Ennes HS, et al. Agonists of proteinase-activated receptor-2 induce inflammation by a neurogenic mechanism. Nature Medicine. 2000;**6**(2):151-158

[9] Cenac N, Garcia-Villar R, Ferrier L, Larauche M, Vergnolle N, Bunnett NW, et al. Proteinase-activated receptor-2-induced colonic inflammation in mice: Possible involvement of afferent neurons, nitric oxide, and paracellular permeability. Journal of Immunology. 2003;**170**(8):4296-4300

[10] Miampamba M, Sharkey KA. Distribution of calcitonin gene-related peptide, somatostatin, substance P and vasoactive intestinal polypeptide in experimental colitis in rats. Neurogastroenterology and Motility. 1998;**10**(4):315-329

[11] Traub RJ, Hutchcroft K, Gebhart GF. The peptide content of colonic afferents decreases following colonic inflammation. Peptides. 1999;**20**(2):267-273

[12] Honore P, Kamp EH, Rogers SD, Gebhart GF, Mantyh PW. Activation of lamina I spinal cord neurons that express the substance P receptor in visceral nociception and hyperalgesia. The Journal of Pain. 2002;**3**(1):3-11

[13] Shah MK, Wan J, Janyaro H, Tahir AH, Cui L, Ding MX. Visceral hypersensitivity is provoked by 2,4,6-trinitrobenzene sulfonic acid-induced ileitis in rats. Frontiers in Pharmacology. 2016;**7**(July):1-13

[14] Wan J, Ding Y, Tahir AH, Shah MK, Janyaro H, Li X, et al. Electroacupuncture attenuates visceral hypersensitivity by inhibiting

JAK2/STAT3 signaling pathway in the descending pain modulation system. Frontiers in Pharmacology. 2017;**11**(Nov):1-15

[15] Shah MK, Ding Y, Wan J, Janyaro H, Tahir AH, Vodyanoy V, et al. Electroacupuncture intervention of visceral hypersensitivity is involved in PAR-2-activation and CGRP-release in the spinal cord. Science Reports. 2020;**10**:11188

[16] Maggi CA. Tachykinins as peripheral modulators of primary afferent nerves and visceral sensitivity. Pharmacological Research. 1997;**36**(2):153-169

[17] Bueno L. Protease-activated receptor-2: A new target for IBS treatment. European Review for Medical and Pharmacological Sciences. 2008;**12**(Suppl. 1):95-102

[18] Plourde V, St-Pierre S, Quirion R. Calcitonin gene-related peptide in viscerosensitive response to colorectal distension in rats. The American Journal of Physiology. 1997;**273**(1 Pt 1):G191-G196

[19] Gschossmann JM, Coutinho SV, Miller JC, Huebel K, Naliboff B, Wong HC, et al. Involvement of spinal calcitonin gene-related peptide in the development of acute visceral hyperalgesia in the rat. Neurogastroenterology and Motility. 2001;**13**(3):229-236

[20] Kong W, McConalogue K, Khitin LM, Hollenberg MD, Payan DG, Böhm SK, et al. Luminal trypsin may regulate enterocytes through proteinase-activated receptor 2. Proceedings of the National Academy of Sciences of the United States of America. 1997;**94**(16):8884-8889

[21] Vergnolle N. Modulation of visceral pain and inflammation by protease-activated receptors. British Journal of Pharmacology. 2004;**141**(8):1264-1274

[22] Liang WJ, Zhang G, Luo HS, Liang LX, Huang D, Zhang FC. Tryptase and protease-activated receptor 2 expression levels in irritable bowel syndrome. Gut Liver. 2016;**10**(3):382-390

[23] Hassler SN, Kume M, Mwirigi JM, Ahmad A, Shiers S, Wangzhou A, et al. The cellular basis of protease activated receptor type 2 (PAR2) evoked mechanical and affective pain. bioRxiv. 2020;**5**(11):1-17

[24] Nystedt S, Ramakrishnan V, Sundelin J. The proteinase-activated receptor 2 is induced by inflammatory mediators in human endothelial cells. Comparison with the thrombin receptor. The Journal of Biological Chemistry. 1996;**271**(25):14910-14915

[25] Cenac N, Coelho AM, Nguyen C, Compton S, Andrade-Gordon P, MacNaughton WK, et al. Induction of intestinal inflammation in mouse by activation of proteinase-activated receptor-2. The American Journal of Pathology. 2002;**161**(5):1903-1915

[26] Nguyen C, Coelho AM, Grady E, Compton SJ, Wallace JL, Hollenberg MD, et al. Colitis induced by proteinase-activated receptor-2 agonists is mediated by a neurogenic mechanism. Canadian Journal of Physiology and Pharmacology. 2003;**81**(9):920-927

[27] Vergnolle N, Ferazzini M, Dandrea MR, Buddenkotte J, Steinhoff M. Proteinase-activated receptors: Novel signals for peripheral nerves. Trends in Neurosciences. 2003;**26**(9):496-500

[28] Lohman RJ, Cotterell AJ, Suen J, Liu L, Do AT, Vesey DA, et al. Antagonism of protease-activated receptor 2 protects against experimental colitis. The Journal of Pharmacology and Experimental Therapeutics. 2012;**340**(2):256-265

[29] Hyun E, Andrade-Gordon P, Steinhoff M, Vergnolle N. Protease-activated receptor-2 activation: A major actor in intestinal inflammation. Gut. 2008;**57**(9):1222-1229

[30] Suckow SK, Caudle RM. NMDA receptor subunit expression and PAR-2 receptor activation in colospinal afferent neurons (CANs) during inflammation induced visceral hypersensitivity. Molecular Pain. 2009;**5**:54

[31] Kim JA, Choi SC, Yun KJ, Kim DK, Han MK, Seo GS, et al. Expression of protease-activated receptor 2 in ulcerative colitis. Inflammatory Bowel Diseases. 2003;**9**(4):224-229

[32] Christerson U, Keita V, Söderholm JD, Gustafson-Svärd C. Increased expression of protease-activated receptor-2 in mucosal mast cells in Crohn's ileitis. Journal of Crohn's & Colitis. 2009;**3**(2):100-108

[33] Christerson U, Keita ÅV, Söderholm JD, Gustafson-Svärd C. Potential role of protease-activated receptor-2-stimulated activation of cytosolic phospholipase A2 in intestinal myofibroblast proliferation: Implications for stricture formation in Crohn's disease. Journal of Crohn's & Colitis. 2009;**3**(1):15-24

[34] Vergnolle N. Clinical relevance of proteinase-activated receptors (PARs) in the gut. Gut. 2005;**54**(6):867-874

[35] Saifeddine M, Al-Ani B, Cheng CH, Wang L, Hollenberg MD. Rat proteinase-activated receptor-2 (PAR-2): cDNA sequence and activity of receptor-derived peptides in gastric and vascular tissue. British Journal of Pharmacology. 1996;**118**(3):521-530

[36] Kawabata A, Kuroda R, Nishikawa H, Kawai K. Modulation by protease-activated receptors of the rat duodenal motility in vitro: Possible mechanisms underlying the evoked contraction and relaxation. British Journal of Pharmacology. 1999;**128**(4):865-872

[37] Corvera CU, Dery O, McConalogue K, Bohm SK, Khitin LM, Caughey GH, et al. Mast cell tryptase regulates rat colonic myocytes through proteinase-activated receptor-2. The Journal of Clinical Investigation. 1997;**100**(6):1383-1393

[38] Kawabata A, Kinoshita M, Nishikawa H, Kuroda R, Nishida M, Araki H, et al. The protease-activated receptor-2 agonist induces gastric mucus secretion and mucosal cytoprotection. The Journal of Clinical Investigation. 2001;**107**(11):1443-1450

[39] Kawabata A, Kawao N, Kuroda R, Tanaka A, Itoh H, Nishikawa H. Peripheral PAR-2 triggers thermal hyperalgesia and nociceptive responses in rats. Neuroreport. 2001;**12**(4):715-719

[40] Bhatt DK, Gupta S, Ploug KB, Jansen-Olesen I, Olesen J. mRNA distribution of CGRP and its receptor components in the trigeminovascular system and other pain related structures in rat brain, and effect of intracerebroventricular administration of CGRP on Fos expression in the TNC. Neuroscience Letters. 2014;**559**:99-104

[41] Hokfelt T, Arvidsson U, Ceccatelli S, Cortes R, Cullheim S, Dagerlind A, et al. Calcitonin gene-related peptide

in the brain, spinal cord, and some peripheral systems. Annals of the New York Academy of Sciences. 1992;**657**(1):119-134

[42] Eftekhari S, Salvatore CA, Calamari A, Kane SA, Tajti J, Edvinsson L. Differential distribution of calcitonin gene-related peptide and its receptor components in the human trigeminal ganglion. Neuroscience. 2010;**169**(2):683-696

[43] Edvinsson L, Eftekhari S, Salvatore CA, Warfvinge K. Cerebellar distribution of calcitonin gene-related peptide (CGRP) and its receptor components calcitonin receptor-like receptor (CLR) and receptor activity modifying protein-1 (RAMP-1) in rat. Molecular and Cellular Neurosciences. 2011;**46**(1):333-339

[44] Sternini C, Anderson K. Calcitonin gene-related peptide-containing neurons supplying the rat digestive system: Differential distribution and expression pattern. SomatosensMotRes. 1992;**9**(1):45-59

[45] Muddhrry PK, Ghatki MA, Spokks RA, Jonhs PM, Pierson AM, Hamid QA, et al. Differential expression of ??-CGRP and ??-CGRP by primary sensory neurons and enteric autonomic neurons of the rat. Neuroscience. 1988;**25**(1):195-205

[46] Eftekhari S, Edvinsson L. Calcitonin gene-related peptide (CGRP) and its receptor components in human and rat spinal trigeminal nucleus and spinal cord at C1-level. BMC Neuroscience. 2011;**12**(1):112-129

[47] Perry MJ, Lawson SN. Differences in expression of oligosaccharides, neuropeptides, carbonic anhydrase and neurofilament in rat primary afferent neurons retrogradely labelled via skin, muscle or visceral nerves. Neuroscience. 1998;**85**(1):293-310

[48] Galeazza M, Garry M, Yost H, Strait K, Hargreaves K, Seybold V. Plasticity in the synthesis and storage of substance-P and calcitonin gene-related peptide in primary afferent neurons during peripheral inflammation. Neuroscience. 1995;**66**(2):443-458

[49] Zhang L, Hoff AO, Wimalawansa SJ, Cote GJ, Gagel RF, Westlund KN. Arthritic calcitonin/alpha calcitonin gene-related peptide knockout mice have reduced nociceptive hypersensitivity. Pain. 2001;**89**(2-3):265-273

[50] Wesselmann U. Neurogenic inflammation and chronic pelvic pain. World Journal of Urology. 2001;**19**(3):180-185

[51] Goadsby PJ. Recent advances in understanding migraine mechanisms, molecules and therapeutics. Trends in Molecular Medicine. 2007;**13**(1):39-44

[52] van Rossum D, Hanisch UK, Quirion R. Neuroanatomical localization, pharmacological characterization and functions of CGRP, related peptides and their receptors. Neuroscience and Biobehavioral Reviews. 1997;**21**(5): 649-678

[53] Sun J, Wu X, Meng Y, Cheng J, Ning H, Peng Y, et al. Electro-acupuncture decreases 5-HT, CGRP and increases NPY in the brain-gut axis in two rat models of Diarrhea-predominant irritable bowel syndrome(D-IBS). BMC Complementary and Alternative Medicine. 2015;**15**(1):340

[54] Sun RQ, Tu YJ, Lawand NB, Yan JY, Lin Q, Willis WD. Calcitonin gene-related peptide receptor activation produces PKA- and PKC-dependent mechanical hyperalgesia

and central sensitization. Journal of Neurophysiology. 2004;**92**(5):2859-2866

[55] Bird GC, Han JS, Fu Y, Adwanikar H, Willis WD, Neugebauer V. Pain-related synaptic plasticity in spinal dorsal horn neurons: Role of CGRP. Molecular Pain. 2006;**2**(1):31

[56] Aich A, Afrin LB, Gupta K. Mast cell-mediated mechanisms of nociception. International Journal of Molecular Sciences. 2015;**16**:29069

[57] Diest SA V, Stanisor OI, Boeckxstaens GE, Jonge WJ De, Wijngaard RMVD. Relevance of mast cell-nerve interactions in intestinal nociception. Biochimica et Biophysica Acta. 2012;**1822**(1):74-84

[58] Kowalski ML, Kaliner MA. Neurogenic inflammation, vascular permeability, and mast cells. Journal of Immunology. 1988;**140**(11):3905-3911

[59] Adam B, Liebregts T, Gschossmann JM, Krippner C, Scholl F, Ruwe M, et al. Severity of mucosal inflammation as a predictor for alterations of visceral sensory function in a rat model. Pain. 2006;**123**(1-2):179-186

[60] Geppetti P, Trevisani M. Activation and sensitisation of the vanilloid receptor: Role in gastrointestinal inflammation and function. British Journal of Pharmacology. 2004;**141**(8):1313-1320

[61] Amadesi S, Nie J, Vergnolle N, Cottrell GS, Grady EF, Trevisani M, et al. Protease-activated receptor-2 sensitizes the capsaicin receptor transient receptor potential vanilloid receptor-1 to induce hyperalgesia. The Journal of Neuroscience. 2004;**24**(18):4300-4312

[62] Grant AD, Cottrell GS, Amadesi S, Trevisani M, Nicoletti P, Materazzi S, et al. Protease-activated receptor-2 sensitizes the transient receptor potential vanilloid-4 ion channel to cause mechanical hyperalgesia in mice. The Journal of Physiology. 2007;**578**(Pt 3):715-733

[63] Murase K, Ryu PD, Randic M. Excitatory and inhibitory amino acids and peptide-induced responses in acutely isolated rat spinal dorsal horn neurons. Neuroscience Letters. 1989;**103**(1):56-63

[64] Humenick AG, Chen BN, Brookes SJH. Gut mechano-nociceptors can be activated by intra-arterial pressure in the physiological range. In: 1st Annual Meeting : Australasian Neuro Gastroenterology & Motility Association Inc (ANGMA). 2014. p. 8

[65] Calam J, Ghatei MA, Domin J, Adrian TE, Myszor M, Gupta S, et al. Regional differences in concentrations of regulatory peptides in human colon mucosal biopsy. Digestive Diseases and Sciences. 1989;**34**(8):1193-1198

[66] Surrenti C, Renzi D, Garcea MR, Surrenti E, Salvadori G. Colonic vasoactive intestinal polypeptide in ulcerative colitis. Journal of Physiology Paris. 1993;**87**(5):307-311

[67] Yamamoto H, Morise K, Kusugami K. Furusawa a, Konagaya T, Nishio Y, et al. Abnormal neuropeptide concentration in rectal mucosa of patients with inflammatory bowel disease. Journal of Gastroenterology. 1996;**31**(4):525-532

[68] Szallasi A, Blumberg PM. Vanilloid (Capsaicin) receptors and mechanisms. Pharmacological Reviews. 1999;**51**(2):159-212

[69] Matsumoto K, Hosoya T, Tashima K, Namiki T, Murayama T, Horie S. Distribution of transient receptor potential vanilloid 1

channel-expressing nerve fibers in mouse rectal and colonic enteric nervous system: Relationship to peptidergic and nitrergic neurons. Neuroscience. 2011;**172**:518-534

[70] Sternini C. Enteric and visceral afferent CGRP neurons. Annals of the New York Academy of Sciences. 1992;**657**(1):170-186

[71] Bueno L, Fioramonti J. Visceral perception: Inflammatory and non-inflammatory mediators. Gut. 2002;**51**(Suppl. 1):i19-i23

[72] Eysselein E, Nast C, Snape J. Calcitonin gene-related peptide and Substance P Decrease in the Rabbit Colon During Colitis A Time Study. Gastroenterology. 1991;**101**(5):1211-1219

[73] Sun YN, Luo JY. Effects of tegaserod on Fos, substance P and calcitonin gene-related peptide expression induced by colon inflammation in lumbarsacral spinal cord. World Journal of Gastroenterology. 2004;**10**(12):1830-1833

[74] Harrington AM, Brierley SM, Isaacs N, Hughes PA, Castro J, Blackshaw LA. Sprouting of colonic afferent central terminals and increased spinal mitogen-activated protein kinase expression in a mouse model of chronic visceral hypersensitivity. The Journal of Comparative Neurology. 2012;**520**(10):2241-2255

[75] Plourde V, Boivin M, St-Pierre S, McDuff J. CGRP plays a role in mediating visceral nociception induced by rectocolonic distension in the rat. Gastroenterology. 1995;**108**(4):A669

[76] Bueno L, Fioramonti J, Delvaux M, Frexinos J. Mediators and pharmacology of visceral sensitivity: From basic to clinical investigations. Gastroenterology. 1997;**112**(5):1714-1743

[77] Chiocchetti R, Grandis A, Bombardi C, Lucchi ML, Dal Lago DT, Bortolami R, et al. Extrinsic and intrinsic sources of calcitonin gene-related peptide immunoreactivity in the lamb ileum: A morphometric and neurochemical investigation. Cell and Tissue Research. 2006;**323**(2):183-196

[78] Coelho AM, Vergnolle N, Guiard B, Fioramonti J, Bueno L. Proteinases and proteinase-activated receptor-2: A possible role to promote visceral hyperalgesia in rats. Gastroenterology. 2002;**122**(4):1035-1047

[79] Cenac N, Chin AC, Garcia-Villar R, Salvador-Cartier C, Ferrier L, Vergnolle N, et al. PAR-2 activation alters colonic paracellular permeability in mice via IFN-gamma-dependent and -independent pathways. The Journal of Physiology. 2004;**558** (Pt 3):913-925

[80] Reed DE, Barajas-Lopez C, Cottrell G, Velazquez-Rocha S, Dery O, Grady EF, et al. Mast cell tryptase and proteinase-activated receptor 2 induce hyperexcitability of guinea-pig submucosal neurons. The Journal of Physiology. 2003;**547**(Pt 2):531-542

[81] Du L, Long Y, Kim JJ, Chen B, Zhu Y, Dai N. Protease activated Receptor-2 induces immune activation and visceral hypersensitivity in post-infectious irritable bowel syndrome mice. Digestive Diseases and Sciences. 2018;**64**(3):729-739

[82] Shi HL, Liu CH, Ding LL, Zheng Y, Fei XY, Lu L, et al. Alterations in serotonin, transient receptor potential channels and protease-activated receptors in rats with irritable bowel syndrome attenuated by Shugan decoction. World Journal of Gastroenterology. 2015;**21**(16):4852-4863

[83] Cenac N, Andrews CN, Holzhausen M, Chapman K, Cottrell G, Andrade-Gordon P, et al. Role for protease activity in visceral pain in irritable bowel syndrome. The Journal of Clinical Investigation. 2007;**117**(3):636-647

[84] Gecse K, Róka R, Ferrier L, Leveque M, Eutamene H, Cartier C, et al. Increased faecal serine protease activity in diarrhoeic IBS patients: A colonic lumenal factor impairing colonic permeability and sensitivity. Gut. 2008;**57**(5):591-599

[85] Annahazi A, Gecse K, Dabek M, Ait-Belgnaoui A, Rosztoczy A, Roka R, et al. Fecal proteases from diarrheic-IBS and ulcerative colitis patients exert opposite effect on visceral sensitivity in mice. Pain. 2009;**144**(1-2):209-217

[86] Tooth D, Garsed K, Singh G, Marciani L, Lam C, Fordham I, et al. Characterisation of faecal protease activity in irritable bowel syndrome with diarrhoea: Origin and effect of gut transit. Gut. 2014;**63**(5):753-760

[87] Vergnolle N, Wallace JL, Bunnett NW, Hollenberg MD. Protease-activated receptors in inflammation, neuronal signaling and pain. Trends in Pharmacological Sciences. 2001;**22**(3):146-152

[88] Kawabata A, Kawao N, Kitano T, Matsunami M, Satoh R, Ishiki T, et al. Colonic hyperalgesia triggered by proteinase-activated receptor-2 in mice: Involvement of endogenous bradykinin. Neuroscience Letters. 2006;**402**(1-2):167-172

[89] Valdez-Morales EE, Overington J, Guerrero-Alba R, Ochoa-Cortes F, Ibeakanma CO, Spreadbury I, et al. Sensitization of peripheral sensory nerves by mediators from colonic biopsies of diarrhea-predominant irritable bowel syndrome patients: A role for PAR2. The American Journal of Gastroenterology. 2013;**108**(10):1634-1643

[90] Xu W, Yuan M, Wu X, Geng H, Chen L, Zhou J, et al. Electroacupuncture relieves visceral hypersensitivity by inactivating protease-activated receptor 2 in a rat model of postinfectious irritable bowel syndrome. Evidence-based Complementary and Alternative Medicine. 2018:7048584

[91] Clark AK, Yip PK, Malcangio M. The liberation of fractalkine in the dorsal horn requires microglial cathepsin S. The Journal of Neuroscience. 2009;**29**(21):6945-6954

[92] Cattaruzza F, Lyo V, Jones E, Pham D, Hawkins J, Kirkwood K, et al. Cathepsin S is activated during colitis and causes visceral hyperalgesia by a PAR 2-dependent mechanism in mice. Gastroenterology. 2011;**141**(5):1864-1874

[93] Fiorucci S, Distrutti E. Role of PAR2 in pain and inflammation. Trends in Pharmacological Sciences. 2002;**23**(4):153-155

[94] Hoogerwerf WA, Zou L, Shenoy M, Sun D, Micci MA, Lee-Hellmich H, et al. The proteinase-activated receptor 2 is involved in nociception. The Journal of Neuroscience. 2001;**21**(22):9036-9042

[95] Hoogerwerf WA, Shenoy M, Winston JH, Xiao SY, He Z, Pasricha PJ. Trypsin mediates nociception via the proteinase-activated receptor 2: A potentially novel role in pancreatic pain. Gastroenterology. 2004;**127**(3):883-891

[96] Wang P, Chen FX, Du C, Li CQ, Yu YB, Zuo XL, et al. Increased production of BDNF in colonic epithelial cells induced by fecal supernatants from diarrheic IBS patients. Scientific Reports. 2015;**5**:10121

[97] Delafoy L, Gelot A, Ardid D, Eschalier A, Bertrand C, Doherty AM, et al. Interactive involvement of brain derived neurotrophic factor, nerve growth factor, and calcitonin gene related peptide in colonic hypersensitivity in the rat. Gut. 2006;**55**(7):940-945

[98] Thompson BJ, Washington MK, Kurre U, Singh M, Rula EY, Emeson RB. Protective roles of alpha-calcitonin and beta-calcitonin gene-related peptide in spontaneous and experimentally induced colitis. Digestive Diseases and Sciences. 2008;**53**(1):229-241

[99] Julia V, Bueno L. Tachykininergic mediation of viscerosensitive responses to acute inflammation in rats: Role of CGRP. The American Journal of Physiology. 1997;**272**(1 Pt 1):G141-G146

[100] Deng D-X, Tan J, Zhang H, Huang G-L, Li S, Guo K-K, et al. Electroacupuncture relieves visceral hypersensitivity by down-regulating mast cell number PAR-2/TRPV 1 signaling, etc. in colonic tissue of rats with irritable bowel syndrome. Acupuncture Research. 2018;**43**(8):485-491

[101] Noor-Mohammadi E, Ligon CO, Mackenzie K, Stratton J, Shnider S, Greenwood-Van MB. A Monoclonal Anti–Calcitonin gene-related peptide antibody decreases stress-induced colonic hypersensitivity. The Journal of Pharmacology and Experimental Therapeutics. 2021;**379**(3):270-279

[102] Zhang L, Song J, Hou X. Mast cells and irritable bowel syndrome: From the bench to the bedside. Journal of Neurogastroenterology and Motility. 2016;**22**(2):181-192

[103] Qiao LY, Grider JR. Colitis induces calcitonin gene-related peptide expression and Akt activation in rat primary afferent pathways. Experimental Neurology. 2009;**219**(1):93-103

Section 2

Female Reproduction Models

Chapter 6

Our Clear-Cut Improvement to the Impact of Mouse and Rat Models in the Research Involving Female Reproduction

Uloma B. Elvis-Offiah, Success Isuman, Marvelous O. Johnson, Vivian G. Ikeh and Sandra Agbontaen

Abstract

In most research involving female reproductive function, female animals particularly mice and rats are usually employed. This may perhaps be due to their well-defined reproductive cycle (estrous cycle) as well as the ability to breed and handle them easily. The short and precise length of estrus cycle usually 4–5 days make mice models the choicest mammal when it comes to human related research. Also, they possess very short reproductive age typically 7–8 months reaching sexual maturity at weeks 4–7 following their birth. Although many similarities exist between this model and humans, however, there also exist obvious distinctions between the human female reproductive system and that of mice. Humans have average length of their reproductive or menstrual cycle of about 28–29 days with their reproductive ages between 10–40 years. These relevant differences between mice and human reproductive system constitute the limitations to the use of this models. Therefore, the scope of this chapter will be to explore the basic knowledge of laboratory mice by examining their reproductive system anatomy and physiology, the fertilization process, estrous cycle and genetic make-up. We hope that this will provide many insights to the use of animal models in female reproductive research.

Keywords: female mice, estrogen and progesterone signaling, female reproductive cycle, estrous cycle, ovary

1. Introduction

The female reproductive system and processes are dynamic in both humans and rodents, undergoing morphological and cytological changes in response to hormonal signals throughout the estrus (for rodent) or menstrual (for human) cycle. These changes are also observed during pregnancy as well as during menopause or ovarian aging. Mice and rats are animals belonging to the Rodentia order and the Muridae family, and so are referred to as murine. Mice and rat models have been established in

IntechOpen

preclinical research involving investigations and assessments of reproductive physiological and pathological processes in humans. Their little size as well as the simplicity of their housing and maintenance allow them to be commonly employed in research. Mice and rats are employed as good models of mammalian pathology and physiology given that the use of people and food animals in studies is hampered by economic and ethical reasons.

In experiments relating to human development, the mice models have been mostly utilized to examine the pathogenesis as well as the general attributes in developmental processes. The ample justification for their relevance to human reproductive tract development and functions lies in their hormone action. Just like in humans, their reproductive cycle oscillates periodically through fluctuations in ovarian steroid concentrations (estrogens and progesterone). There also exist these steroid hormone receptors (ER, PR) systems in some of their reproductive organs like the uterus and mammary glands which act as controls to check hormone levels and translate the info into suitable developmental effects. They possess similar reproductive cycle phases as humans. Their reproductive cycle is divided into two developmental phases: the preparatory phase, which is evidenced by high estrogen and progesterone concentrations and occurs throughout proestrus stage. During estrus, this phase leaves the ovarian target tissues prepared for gestation. The second phase occurs in diestrus when progesterone levels drop, and it is characterized by the apoptotic elimination of previous arrangements.

In order to uncover human developmental pathways and gain insight into female reproductive behaviors, developmental scientists have used a number of animals to explore the morphogenetic and molecular mechanisms involved in vertebrate development [1]. Organogenesis and differentiation have been studied extensively in embryonic, fetal, and neonatal mice and rats, with the unspoken assumption that morphogenetic and molecular processes in mice are equivalent to those in humans. This argument is supported by the fact that mice and humans share many developmental features. With a few exceptions, both species share the same range of organs and developmental phases that appear to be equivalent, if not identical [2, 3].

Whereas the data above illustrate that mice research is important to human reproductive biology, the mouse and human reproductive systems have distinct morphogenetic, physiologic, and anatomical distinctions. The lack of information on human organogenesis, particularly in terms of molecular pathways, makes human/mouse comparisons challenging.

1.1 Comparison of the basic anatomy of the reproductive organs of the female mice to humans

The female mice reproductive systems are made up of two ovaries, two small tightly coiled uterine tubes, two uterine horns, the cervix and the vaginal canal (**Figure 1**). The vagina is a tiny gray tube that connects the bladder to the uterus. In mice, the Mullerian ducts start at the opening of the uterine tube and develop into the female genital tract while in the rats, the ovarian bursa is formed when the ostium forms a complete capsule around the ovary. The uterine horns divide the vagina and reach toward the kidneys. Both the mice and rats possess bicornuate uterus which may accommodate several embryos known as litters. On the other hand, women have simple uterus which have only one compartment for the development of one or two embryo(s) (**Figure 1**). Ovaries in humans are little lumpy glands that sit at the terminals of the uterine horns and are connected to the uterine horns by oviducts.

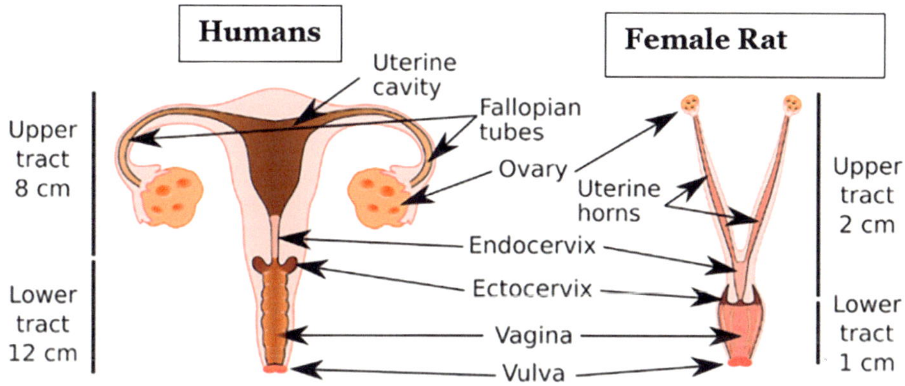

Figure 1.
Anatomical feature of the reproductive system of a female rat and human.

1.1.1 Mice uterus and cervix in comparison with humans

The human uterus is simplex and appears in form of a large pear-like shape with a unique cavity which measures about 8 cm when assessing it from one cornu to the other cornu and 5 cm in width (**Figure 1**). Nevertheless, steroid hormone levels as well as pregnancy status extensively determines the thickness of the uterus. Other factors that affect uterus thickness include the existence of leiomyomata. On the other hand, mouse uterus is bicornuate having two cornua that unite distally to create a singular body (corpus), but in rats, the uterus is duplex, with twin uterine horns that are partially linked at the caudal end. A part of the broad ligament known as mesometria suspend the mouse uterus horns from the dorsal wall and hold them in place. These ligaments encircle the blood and lymphatic vessels as well as many nerves. Similarly, from the lateral pelvic side walls, the human uterus is also suspended by comparable ligaments. The body of the uterus both in humans and mice is made up of the caudal-cervical and cranial-fundal sections. The caudal-cervical and cranial-fundal regions of the uterus are also found in mice. However, the cranial portion of the body of mouse uterus is separated by a median septum into two chambers. On the other hand, rat uterus is partly connected and has no complete body. Nonetheless, it has a unique cervix with two uterine horn canals that are distinct. Both dorsally and ventrally, mice and rats have a continuous cervix and vaginal walls but not laterally. The lateral vaginal walls continue on both sides forming deep fornices. But then, in humans, the cervix (ectocervical portion) protrudes into the vaginal canal, having wide posterior and anterior fornices and thinner lateral fornices.

1.1.2 Comparison of the oviduct (uterine tube)

The oviduct, generally termed the uterine tube in mice and rats is a complex tiny-curled tube that links to the periovarian area. The mesotubarium helps to suspend the oviduct to the dorsal body wall, and is connected to the mesovarium, uterine mesometrium and ovarian bursa. Whereas the human oviduct is a muscle-lined straight tube that is about 12 cm long. The human oviduct, like that of rodents, is connected to the respective ovary by a broad ligament that runs from the uterine cornu (horn) (**Table 1**). In both the mice, rat and human oviducts are found the intramuscular segment, the isthmus, the ampulla, the infundibulum, and a fimbriated terminal [4].

Feature	Rodent (rat and mice)	Human
Gross anatomy		
Ovary	Sphere-shaped and contained in bursa	Oval-shaped and opened to peritoneal cavity
Uterine tube	Thin tightly coiled tube, 18–30 mm in length	Muscle-lined straight tube, 12 cm in length
Uterine tube association to ovary	Open immediately into the ovarian bursa	Fimbriated end of the ampulla opens immediately into peritoneal cavity near the ovary
Segments of uterine tube	Ampulla, infundibulum and intramural	Like rodents
Type of uterus	Rat: has duplex and bicornuate uterus having double lateral horns. Mouse: Bicornuate uterus possessing dual lateral horns and a one body.	Simplex uterus
Histology		
Type of epithelium in the oviduct	Ampulla segment diffusely ciliated	Scattered peg cells and simple ciliated columnar cells
Number of ciliated cells	Reduces as the uterine tube move towards the uterus	The ampulla and infundibulum have a large number of ciliated cells, but the intramural portion has a smaller number
Myometrium	Outer longitudinal and Inner circular smooth muscle coats	Single smooth muscular layer
Myometrial glands	Mouse: incidence differs by strain rat: absent	Absent

Table 1.
Comparison of the female reproductive system of rat and human.

Inside the uterine wall is found the oviduct's intramuscular section which continues into the dorsolateral side of uterus wall in rodents, forming the colliculus tubarius, a modest extension into the uterine cavity. The dimension of this extension differs although it is usually a smaller number (1mm in length). Depending on uterine size, the human oviduct's intramuscular section length varies and reaches laterally from the superior corner of the cornu until it arises from the uterus wall. A brief segment of the oviduct, the isthmus runs laterally from the uterus wall to the ampulla (**Figure 1**). This segment is significantly more firmly twisted in mice than in humans [5]. The ampulla is a dilated section that connects the oviduct's infundibulum to the isthmus. From the infundibulum, the oviduct of mice grows a fimbriated side that emerges into periovarian area and the peritoneal cavity close to the ovary. In humans, one of these fimbriae joins the ovary to the oviduct.

1.2 Sexual maturation in female murine (rat and mice) compared to humans

In adult female mice, reproduction is comprised of a sequence of neurological and hormonal changes that interact to allow the creation of offspring. The connection between the anterior pituitary and ovarian hormones, as well as placental hormones, is involved in this process (during pregnancy). The hypothalamus, in particular, plays a key role in controlling the anterior pituitary's ability to manufacture and secrete gonadotropin hormones (Follicle stimulating hormone, FSH and Luteinizing hormone, LH). FSH enhances the development of gametes in both male and female animals, whereas LH stimulates the release of estrogen and progesterone (gonadal hormones) in females as well as androgen in males. Lactation is regulated by prolactin, an anterior pituitary hormone.

Secondary sexual traits and the correct functioning of the genital tract are maintained by gonadal hormones, that also work somewhat on central nervous system to ensure effective coupling [6]. Each part develops at a varying rate, and normal sexual maturity in rats relies on a complex and poorly known interaction among them all.

Sexual maturity normally correlates with increasing circulating gonadotropin titers after 4 weeks of age. In contrast to humans, the specific moment at which maturity occurs is quite varied, therefore such a comment must be interpreted in the context of the measurement used to determine when "sexual maturity" has been attained (**Tables 2** and **3**). Vaginal introitus and a cornified vaginal smear, both estrogen-dependent, are the earliest detectable indications of puberty in mice and rats. Other markers of sexual maturity, such as mate readiness, the capacity to conceive and carry a litter to term, and maybe sexual maturity as measured by the ability to produce weanling-age young, have a more convoluted hormonal foundation. The vaginal opening can happen as early as day 26 and is usually complete by the 7th weeks (**Tables 2** and **3**). The first vaginal cornification occurs between 24 to 120 hours after the vaginal opening has been created, however this is very variable. Furthermore, estrus (the urge to mate) does not always occur on a regular timetable, which can contribute to unpredictability and make it difficult to use as an experimental tool.

Regardless of how it is measured, the process of achieving sexual maturity is a very varied one. According to the timing of vaginal opening, inbred mice strains generally mature by 7 weeks of age, however some researchers have observed a median age of 35 days and a range of 26 to 49 days in C57BL/6 and BALB/c strains [7]. Vaginal opening has been discovered as early as 24 days in certain experimental animals. Two key drivers to such variety are genetic background and season. Many studies have discovered

Feature	Rodent (rat and mice)	Human
Puberty		
Age at onset	Mouse: Approximately 4 weeks rat: 26–49 days	Almost 10–11 years, continuing for 4 years
Estradiol production by ovaries	Effect varies with strains	Causes breast and uterus development as well as pubertal developmental surge and closure of epiphyseal plate
Exposure of immature females to male urine	Can hasten puberty	Not studied
Exposure of immature females to urine from group-housed females	Mouse: be able to slow down puberty Rat: undetermined	Not studied
Day length and temperature	Be able to affect puberty	No effect

Table 2.
Sexual maturity and ovulation in rat and human.

Feature	Endometrial phase	Mice and rats	Human
Proestrus	Proliferative	Distended and hyperemic with mitotic epithelium and presence of leukocytic stroma	Glands of tubular shapes with columnar epithelial cells. Mitotic glands and stroma
Estrus	Secretory	Full mitoses, little or no leukocytes	Columnar epithelium; more tortuous and distended glands, subnuclear vacuoles in cells at the beginning of secretory phase, after which supranuclear vacuoles followed by ultimate disappearance of the vacuoles. Under the effect of progesterone, gradually increasing epithelioid stroma ensues through the last part of the secretory phase
Metestrus	Shedding	Degenerated epithelium, uterine wall collapse, elevated amounts of leukocytes	Condensed stroma; neutrophilic infiltration and epithelial disintegration
Diestrus	Early proliferative	Uterus collapses with high leukocytes and redevelopment	Lacking

Table 3.
Difference between human endometrial cycle and mouse estrous cycle.

that there is some inter-strain variability. For example, Drake et al. [8] discovered that vaginal introitus occurs at a younger age in the summer than in the winter. He was able to account for a considerable percentage of the linked variation by matching a sine curve to the data and accounting for seasonal fluctuations. The season of the year also has a huge impact. Experimental exposure to cold delays vaginal opening, the first cornified smear, and the first typical estrus.

1.3 Relationship between menstrual cycle and estrous cycle

The menstrual cycle, as well as the estrus cycle, is controlled by the regular intermittent fluctuations in the mean value of estradiol (E2) and progesterone (P4) gonadal steroid hormones in endocrine fashion (**Figure 2**). In tissues such as the uterus and ovaries, E2 and P4 receptors (ER, PR) track the concentrations of these hormones and convert the information into timed developmental feedbacks.

The key integrator of both the menstrual and estrous cycles is gonadotropin releasing hormone (GnRH), a neurohormone discharged in pulsatile manner by the hypothalamus. The GnRH, when released is transported via the hypophyseal tract to the anterior pituitary gland that causes the production of FSH and LH gonadotropic hormones (**Figure 3**). These hormones are conveyed in the blood vessels to the ovaries to cause development of follicles and resultant production of E2. In this regard, FSH has stronger effects. During the pre-ovulatory stage, E2 confers a positive feedback effect on GnRH, FSH and LH production thereby increasing its own concentration, while it elicits a negative feedback effect during the post-ovulation period [9].

Two contrasting developmental phases exist in both menstrual and estrous cycles. The first is the follicular phase (in humans) also known as pro-estrus phase (in animals). It is a preparatory stage evident by the raised E2 and P4 levels (**Figures 2** and **4**). These steroid hormones initiate the proliferation of the endometrium and growth of

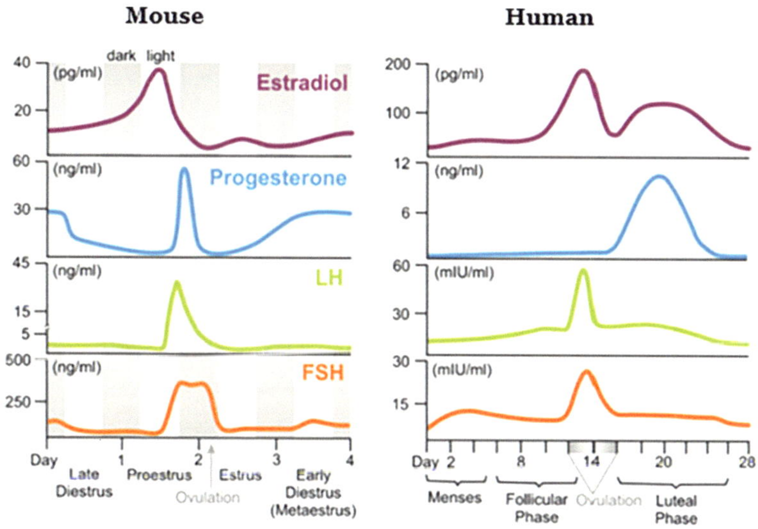

Figure 2.
The 4–6 day mouse reproductive cycle (left panel) is compared to the 28-day human menstrual cycle (right panel). In this diagram, average fluctuations of estradiol, progesterone, LH, and FSH (Maeda et al., 2000).

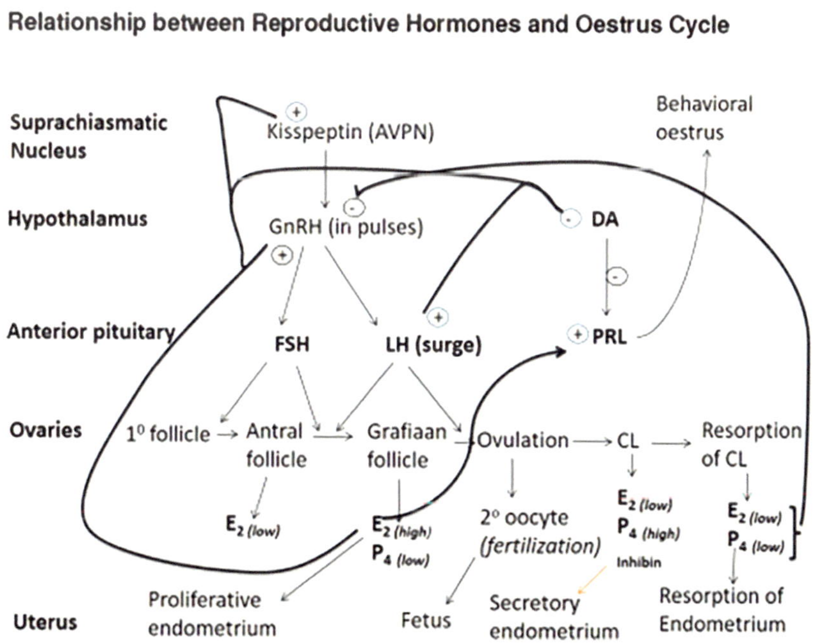

Figure 3.
Activities of reproductive hormones on the ovaries in estrus phase. The hypothalamus through E_2 positive feedback loop secretes GnRH which consequently increases FSH concentration. The FSH reaches the ovaries to cause the development of the follicles which secrets E_2. The increased E_2 levels cause the proliferation of endometrial lining and inhibition of DA. The inhibition of DA releases PRL from DA suppression. PRL maintains CL formed after ovulation. After ovulation, E_2 confer a negative feedback effect on the secretion of GnRH, FSH and LH. CL formed produces high concentrations of P_4 and low E_2 levels leading to secretory activity in oviduct and endometrium. The low E_2 concentration releases the GnRH and DA from inhibition. DA suppresses PRL leading to CL regression and consequent low levels of P_4. GnRH = gonadotropin releasing hormone, LH = luteinizing hormone, FSH = follicle stimulating hormone, P_4 = progesterone, E_2 = estrogen, PRL = prolactin, DA = dopamine and CL = corpus luteum.

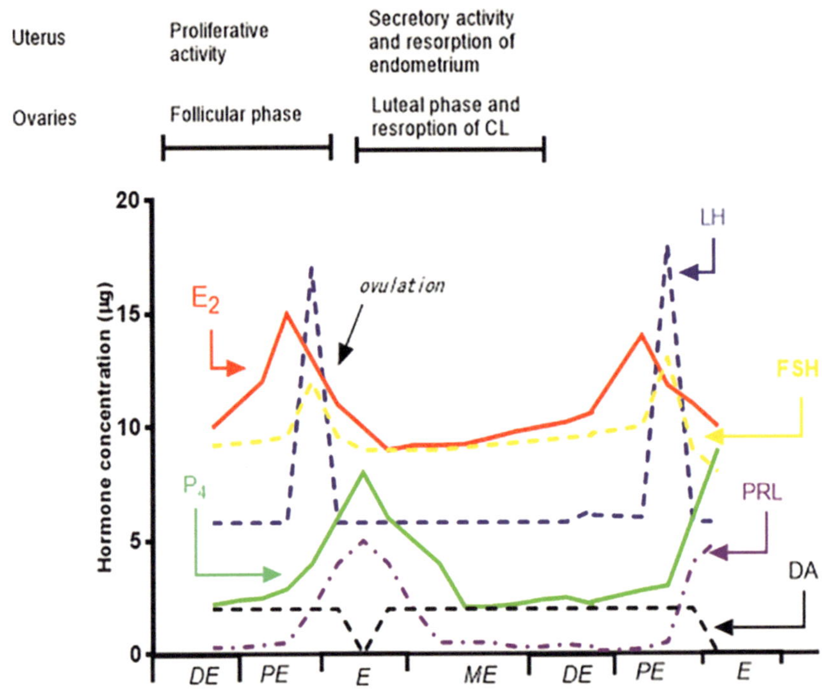

Figure 4.
The hormonal levels in each phase of mouse reproductive cycle. Diestrus is the end of luteal phase; pro-estrus is the beginning of follicular phase. DE = diestrus, PE = pro-estrus, E = estrus, ME = metestrus, GnRH = gonadotropin releasing hormone, E_2 = estradiol, P_4 = progesterone, PRL = prolactin, DA = Dopamine, LH = luteinizing hormone, FSH = Follicle stimulating hormone.

blood vessels and prime the reproductive tissues for pregnancy [10]. The second is the luteal phase (in humans) also identified as metestrus phase (in animals). It begins as E2 and P4 concentrations decline and manifests as apoptotic breaking up of the former preparations in addition to resorption of the uterine endometrium. The most outstanding peculiarity of the estrous cycle is the steady E2 surge in late diestrus to pro-estrus. This event marks the border between the two developmental phases of the cycle and signifies the beginning of a fresh cycle [11].

1.4 Difference between menstrual cycle and estrous cycle

Mice and rats go through estrous cycles, of which if fertilization failed to occur during the cycle, resorption of endometrium occurs. Humans on the other hand, experience menstrual cycle of which their endometrium is shed during the course of menstruation if fertilization and conception failed to occur. One more difference is in their sexual behavior during ovulation [12]. Female mice and rats are normally sexually receptive and active solely at some point in their estrous cycle such as during late proestrus and in estrus phase which are the phases where ovulation occurs. This is known and referred to as "heat period." Females of species with menstrual cycle, such as humans, on the other hand, can be sexually receptive and active all over the course of their cycle. Humans also undergo covert ovulation with no visible outside displays of sexual receptivity unlike the mice. Rats, on the contrary frequently display unmistakable outward receptivity to demonstrate estral receptivity at ovulation [13].

A classic menstrual cycle in humans lasts about 28 days, with ovulation taking place at 14th day (**Figure 2**). The estrus cycle is considerably shorter than the menstrual cycle, occurring within 4 to 6 days [14, 15].

Additional key difference between the cycles, aside the overall period necessary for a full cycle, remains that the E2 and P4 peaks are classically disconnected in human menstrual cycle, while they intersect in rodent estrous cycle at the pro-estrus phase [16]. Rodents are furthermore disposed to estrous cycle interference from sensitivity to external or environmental cues such as light, temperature, stress and other factors than the humans are [17].

1.5 The mouse estrous cycle and hormonal changes

Hormonal changes always and frequently manifest as regular alterations in the morphology and cytology of the animal's reproductive tract.

The estrus cycle in mice is divided into 4 distinctive phases – pro-estrus, estrus, metestrus and diestrus. The pro-estrus phase corresponds to follicular phase in humans. At about midday of the beginning of the pro-estrus phase, there exists a significant surge of estradiol (E2) triggering a fast peaking of the LH and FSH in the evening of pro-estrus and an increased progesterone (P4) secretion [11]. As in humans, the gonadotropin surge prompts ovulation and subsequent formation of corpus luteum. This high concentration of E2 inhibits dopamine (DA) and simultaneously increases the concentration of prolactin (PRL) by relieving it from dopamine inhibition (**Figure 3**). All hormones come back to starting levels when ovulation occurs in estrus.

The PRL and P4 levels increase markedly at the early post-ovulation phase (i.e. late estrus) and drops abruptly in metestrus phase (**Figure 4**). The PRL is responsible in maintaining the corpus luteum. During the estrus and metestrus phases, the corpus luteum secretes P4 and to a lesser extent E2 as well as inhibin [14]. All these hormones have combined negative feedback on the GnRH, FSH and LH [9]. By the late diestrus phase, the corpus luteum regresses due to decrease in PRL levels. This effect consequently leads to a decline in E2, P4 and inhibin levels. All these releases the hypothalamus and anterior pituitary from the negative feedback effects of these hormones [11] and initiates the start of a new phase

1.6 Characterization of menstrual cycle using different phases of estrous cycle

1.6.1 Pro-estrus phase

Pro-estrus phase lasts for 24 hours (approximately 1 day) in mice and rats [15]. This phase parallels the pre-ovulatory day of menstrual cycle. For example, E2 concentration rises and confers a positive feedback mechanism on GnRH release. At mid pro-estrus phase, E2 concentration reaches its peak to induce the LH and the FSH surge resulting in ovulation while it confers an inhibitory effect on DA to release PRL suppression [17]. During this phase, P4 and PRL levels begin to rise (**Figure 4**). One or several follicles of the ovaries start(s) to grow and mature (**Figure 3**).

The main characteristics of vaginal cytology of this phase is the existence of large or small, rounded epithelial cells that may be nucleated or enucleated. The cells are fairly of uniform appearance and size. They are usually seen in cohesive sheets, clusters, or strands. The appearance might sometimes not be observed particularly in hypocellularity samples, therefore should not be taken as a yardstick in determining pro-estrus. Sometimes no leucocytes will be seen, however, leucocytes can be found in early pro-estrus.

Moderately low amounts of large epithelial cells plus cornified cells may as well be detected. As the cycle nears estrus, abundant cornified cells will be present (**Table 4**). The presence of high amounts of cornified cells or low numbers of leucocytes should not impede the identification of pro-estrus especially when the usual features of the smear are the small, round epithelial cell population. There might be presence of the secretion in the smear. Visual observation of the vulva will reveal wide opened vagina which will be moist, and the tissues appears deep pink or red. Striations will be seen in both the ventral and dorsal lips of the vulva. The lips may appear swollen.

1.6.2 Estrus phase

Estrous phase lasts between 12 - 48 hours (approximately 2 day) and signifies the beginning of the luteal period in humans [18, 19]. Estrus is the stage when the female mice remain sexually receptive ("on heat" or "in heat"). Under regulation of gonadotropic hormones, estrogen secretions exert their biggest influence. Throughout the morning of estrus E2 levels remains elevated conferring inhibitory effect on DA. The action of high E2 on DA releases PRL from DA suppression. PRL is important in maintenance of CL after ovulation. During the afternoon, E2 falls back to basal levels and the P4 concentration on the other hand rises and peaks (**Figures 3** and **4**). The P4 concentration is important for the secretory activities in the endometrium. The high level of P4 with corresponding low concentrations of E2 inhibits GnRH and FSH and releases the DA from suppression (**Figure 4**). DA then inhibits the PRL causing CL to regress which in turn decreases the concentration of P4 at late estrus.

This phase is typically recognized by the presence of abundant cornified squamous cells. These cells appear in clusters and are of irregular shapes. They have no visible nucleus, and their cytoplasm looks granular. Abundant bacterial cells may be seen. The bacterial cells may stick to the cells or appear freely in the background of the smear. During early and mid-estrus phase, no leucocytes are observed however, can be seen during late phase. There will be predominance of cornified cells (75%) with epithelial cells (<25%) (**Table 4**). Cells can appear in clusters or scattered. During physical visual inspection, the vagina will appear similar to pro-estrus, but it will be less pink or red, less moist but striations might be very prominent for some animals. The vulva lips will be swollen.

1.6.3 Metestrus phase

Metestrus phase marks the mid of luteal phase (post-ovulation) in humans. During this phase, the signs of E2 and P4 stimulation subside. The decline in the plasma levels of P4 stimulates the hypothalamus to secrete GnRH and consequently the gonadotropic hormone, FSH. The FSH in the ovaries starts the development of preantral follicle which secretes E2 (**Figures 3** and **4**). The Low levels of P4 also lead to resorption of endometrial lining. This phase typically is brief occurring within 24 hours [18] or may last for 1–3 days [16], personal experience in our lab, data not published. In this stage, there is presence of leucocytes in combination with few

Cycle phase	Duration (h)	Behavior	Vaginal smear morphology
Proestrus	14	At the end of this phase male acceptance start	Mostly nucleated and non-nucleated epithelial cells (75%) present
Estrus	25–27	Lordosis; sexually receptive	75% cornified cells; 25% nucleated and non-nucleated epithelial cells
Metestrus	21	Not sexually receptive	Many leukocytes (50%) with nucleated and cornified cells
Diestrus	55–57	No male acceptance	Leukocytes (85–100%)
Cycle phases			

Table 4.
Vaginal smear cytology and mice behavior during estrous.

cornified squamous epithelial cells (**Table 4**). In early metestrus, leucocytes are sometimes interspersed or may be tightly clumped together around the cornified cells; the leukocyte cells may equal the quantity of the cornified cells or may be less. At mid-metestrus, leucocytes become higher in number than the cornified cells [14] and the smear might be extremely dense and cellular. By late metestrus, the number of cornified cells decreases with a correspondingly reduction in smear cellularity displaying conversion to diestrus phase. Visual observation of the vulva is characterized by pale coloration. The vaginal canal will be completely sealed and dry. It may additionally be sloughed with white cellular debris.

1.6.4 Diestrus phase

This phase marks the boundary between luteal phase and follicular phase and lasts between 55–57 hours (approximately 3 days) (**Table 4**). If pregnancy fails to occur, the diestrus stage ends with the recession of the CL. In the late stage of diestrus, the hypothalamus through E2 positive feedback loop secretes GnRH and consequently FSH (**Figures 3** and **4**). The FSH in the ovaries causes the development of the follicles from preantral follicle to early Graffian follicle which secretes E2. The increased E2 levels cause the endometrial lining to begin to proliferate. The vaginal cells consist predominantly of leucocytes at the early phase and with nucleated cells but no cornified cells at the late phase. Visual observation will reveal vaginal opening which may be actually moist. The orifice will be slightly opened or totally closed in some animal. There will be no tissue swelling or striation.

1.7 Importance of rodent (mice and rats) in research

Because better molecular tools to modify the mouse genome were available in the past, the mouse was frequently used instead of the rat. Recent improvements in genetic methods for creating knockout rat models promise to break down these obstacles, potentially allowing rats to be used in a wider range of scientific studies. In the end, the rodent model of choice is determined by which species best mimics the symptoms and illness process seen in humans. It's evident that rats aren't just big mice, and that each species has advantages and disadvantages that vary depending on the process or gene under investigation. It is very important to adopt the right paradigm for translational medicine because a lot of money is spent exploring medications and cures that ultimately fail at various levels of pre-clinical and clinical trials. One explanation for this is that animal trial results do not always correctly represent human outcomes.

1.8 Limitation of mice as an ideal model of human physiology and disease

When comparing mice and humans, there are several variances in developmental timing and reproductive organ shape, as well as discrepancies in their metabolism. Poly-ovulation and a brief period of gestation period in mice, for example, are important variations from humans. Unlike humans, mice are multiparous species such that exposure to endocrine disrupting compounds during gestation has complicated effects on the offspring. Morley-Fletcher and colleagues [20] showed that during sexual differentiation, exposure to sex steroids gave varied results relative to hormone exchange between the female and male fetuses in mice uterine horns.

There are further differences in reproductive function to consider when comparing humans to other mammals like mice. Human oogenesis determinants, for example, are far more intricate than those of most other mammalian species, including mice. When it comes to studying human reproductive disorders, rodent species/strains have several important limitations. Except in rare strains with certain genetic backgrounds, there are still no germ cell tumors (primary ovarian tumors) in the ovaries of mice or rats; yet it is a common human malignancy in young adult females [21]. It's also worth noting that the outcomes responsive to the effect of repro-toxicants differ amongst mice and rat strains even within the same species. In responding to in utero exposure to a particular phthalate (dibutyl phthalate (DBP)), Wistar rats show elevated incidence of cryptorchidism and reduced rates of epididymal hypoplasia than Sprague-Dawley rats [21].

1.9 Criteria for estrous cycle staging

Changes in estrous cycle can only be effectively predicted and identified if the investigator is adequately acquainted of the continuous variations and appearance in the vaginal cytology throughout the several stages of the animal's reproductive cycle (**Table 5**). There are numerous reports on the appearance of normal reproductive tract of all the different phases of the estrous cycle [14, 16], nevertheless, to attain consistency in method of staging the cycle, the following criteria should be followed.

1. To clarify the interval as well as the stages of the reproductive cycle, cytological samples of the vaginal cells should be collected for a minimum of 14 successive days (can also be done for up to 19 or 21 days). It has to be prepared at a particular time of the day preferably in the early periods of the morning between 7 am and 12 noon [15]. This is vital as Certain short phases may be "missed" particularly if samples are not consistently gathered for instance, in smears harvested too late or very early in the day, pro-estrus phase might be missed. Irrespective of what time the samples are harvested, they must be prepared at about same matching period of the day. This must be maintained throughout the collection

	Mice and rats	Humans
Length	Roughly 4–6 days of estrous cycles except when disrupted by pregnancy	About 28 days
Onset	Starts between 21–26 days after birth	Starts at puberty (10–13 years old) until menopause (40–50 years)
Phases	Metestrus, diestrus, proestrus and estrus,	Proliferative (follicular) Menstruation, and secretory (luteal)
Follicle development/ cycle	Numerous follicles mature concurrently	Several follicles (1–12) start developing, only one or two follicle(s) become(s) dominant
Ova released at ovulation	Multiple	Normally one or two ova per menstrual cycle

Table 5.
Similarities and differences in estrous cycle in mice and ovarian cycle in humans.

period to diminish inconsistency. Vaginal lavage method is ideal for collection of the samples.

2. The typical interval of the estrous cycle is commonly between 4–6 days for 60%–70% of the sample population. However, some animals may present longer regular or irregular cycles.

3. A mouse is considered as cycling regularly, when it presents at least two repeated cycles of the same interval within the 14 days. In other cases, cycling can be determined by checking if estrus immediately follows pro-estrus [22]. This should be the case when ascertaining cycling in mice as they exhibit more varied cycling patterns and can lead to erroneous conclusions.

4. Two repetitive cycles with 1–2 days of estrus, 1 day of metestrus, 1 day of pro-estrus or any with only a day of estrus and 2 to 3 successive days of diestrus in each cycle will also be considered regular.

5. Cycles will be considered 'extended' if there is 4–5 days of estrus or 4–5 days of diestrus.

6. Irregularities in cycle length or cycle contiguity is greater in mice than rats i.e., 4 days followed by 5 days instead of 4 days and vice versa [23, 24] although irregular cycles are predominant with aged animals (6 months and above).

7. Cycles, in which the alternations between the phases do not follow the sequence pro-estrus to estrous specifically, will be considered irregular. They may not necessarily follow the consistent pattern of Pro-estrus, estrous, metestrus and diestrus to conclude as regular. This position is especially advised for mice. Irregular cycles may be characterized by placing them in one group (or they may be excluded from the experiment).

8. Animals that are pseudo-pregnant before administration should be eliminated from the experimental protocol. Such animals will exhibit persistent estrous or

diestrus. Constant light causes persistent estrus and failure to cycle while housing in large groups causes persistent diestrus [25]. Nonetheless, mice in persistent diestrus will synchronize upon exposure to male urine.

9. If the outcome of drug or extract/compound expression on the cycle is even in a set (e.g., consequential persistent diestrus or estrous), so this may provide a valuable summary of the data. Conversely, if some animals exposed to the compound or extract display persistent diestrus, while others exhibit prolonged estrous, then such outcomes may possibly not reveal the alterations caused by the test compound. Therefore, the discrepancy in collection may perhaps result in a general belief that reproductive cycle remained unaffected. The procedure should be repeated in such cases.

1.9.1 Vaginal lavage or smear protocol

The vaginal smear technique for describing the phases of the estrous cycle was initially probed in 1917 by Stockard and Papanicolaou [26, 27]. A slight adjustment of the method is implemented for this procedure, but it essentially involves the recognition of the cell categories and their relative amounts existing in the sample gotten from flushing walls of the vagina. Ascriptions of the features to explicit phases of the estrous cycle were attributed and recorded by Elvis-Offiah and Bafor [28].

1.9.1.1 Preparations

1. Normal saline: use normal saline for intravenous drips or weigh 0.9 g of NaCl (MW 58.44) powder and dissolve in 100 mL distilled water. Thereafter, stocked in a securely air- and watertight vessel at room temperature till required.

2. Slides: clean and label the glass slides according to animal's number and groups.

3. Methanol: Cold 100% methanol is recommended for fixing cells. Though 95% ethanol from absolute ethanol (≥99.8% GC) can also be used. It can be prepared by measuring 95 ml of absolute ethanol into a calibrated cylinder and adding 5 mL of distilled water to make it up to 100 mL.

4. Stains: monochromatic stains are recommended. These include Wright-Giemsa stain, methylene blue, eosin, and crystal violet (5%). For RHERG, we will be using methylene blue/eosin staining. Prepare 0.1% methylene blue in a separate bottle and 0.1% eosin is also prepared separately.

1.9.1.2 Collecting vaginal cells (vaginal lavage)

1. Vaginal smears should be steadily collected daily between 9 am and 12 noon by washing out the vaginal epithelium with normal saline using a disposable Pasteur pipette. The tips of the pipette to be used must compulsorily be even and pointed with an endorsed inner tip bore of ≥1.5 mm for pipette tips (OECD n.d.) [29]. The practice of using a new dropper or tip for each animal is best. Should a lone dropper or tip be employed on different animals, it

must be meticulously cleaned with fresh sterile or distilled water. Thorough cleaning is appropriate to avoid sample contamination between animals which may result in erroneousness staging or, occasionally, reproductive tract infection.

2. Draw around 0.2 mL (rats) or 0.1 mL (mice) of saline water into the dropper or pipette.

3. Pick up the animal from the cage to the cage lid (hopper) with its rear end placed in your direction. Grasp the tail firmly and raise the hind feet. The animal will use merely her forelimbs to grasp the hopper. On the spot, urination may ensue. If so, pause till urination ends. It is advised to clean the vaginal orifice with the saline and with a different tip should urine is left at the vaginal canal opening.

4. The dropper tip should be carefully and softly inserted without penetration into the vaginal opening. At that point, the vaginal wall should be flushed with the saline 2 or 3 times. Draw little amount of vaginal fluid out. If the fluid is milky at the initial draw, then successive flushing is not needed (OECD n.d.) [29]. Inserting the tip too deep into the vaginal orifice may stimulate the cervix to induce pseudo pregnancy therefore care must be taken. Pseudo pregnancy may appear as persistent diestrus or estrus for up to 14 days [11].

5. Gently transfer the fluid comprising the cells on a clean, pre-labelled glass slide bearing the appropriate animal's identity.

6. Allow the smears to air dry then fix with 100% cold methanol for 5–10 minutes on the laboratory bench and allow to dry. Drying can be done by air-drying or by placing on heated surface set at 50°C.

7. Add one-two drops of methylene blue (0.1%) on the slide for 3 minutes. Remove surplus stain by placing a piece of filter paper, cotton wool or any absorbent for a second. Afterward, add 2 drops of eosin (1%) on the slide for 2 minutes. All work must be carried out at room temperature. Avoid heavy staining.

8. Rinse the slide briefly and appropriately with small amount of tap water and keep in standing position to dry.

9. View the slides under light microscope starting from the least eyepiece magnification. Koehler illumination: this gives optimal resolution and contrast [30].

2. Conclusion

Both in humans and rats, the female reproductive system and processes are dynamic, changing morphologically and cytologically in response to hormonal cues during the course of the estrus or monthly cycle. Along with menopause and ovarian age, these changes are also seen during pregnancy. For preclinical evaluations of human reproductive physiological and pathological processes, mice and rats are ideal models. They are frequently used in research due to their small size, simplicity of housing, and maintenance requirements. Their reproductive cycle oscillates periodically because to variations in ovarian steroid concentrations, just like in humans (estrogens and progesterone). However, there are morphogenetic, physiological, and anatomical differences between the mouse and human reproductive systems.

Author details

Uloma B. Elvis-Offiah[1,2]*, Success Isuman[1], Marvelous O. Johnson[1], Vivian G. Ikeh[1] and Sandra Agbontaen[1,3]

1 Faculty of Life Sciences, Department of Science Laboratory Technology, University of Benin, Benin City, Edo State, Nigeria

2 Department of Physiology, College of Medicine, University of Arizona, Tucson, AZ, United State of America

3 Department of Nursing, University of Northampton, Northampton, England, United Kingdom

*Address all correspondence to: uloma.achilihu@uniben.edu

References

[1] Cunha GR, Liu G, Sinclair A, Cao M, Baskin L. Mouse clitoral development and comparison to human clitoral development. Differentiation. 2020;**111**:79-97. DOI: 10.1016/j.diff.2019.07.006

[2] Walters KA, Simanainen U, Handelsman DJ. Molecular insights into androgen actions in male and female reproductive function from androgen receptor knockout models. Human Reproduction Update. 2010;**16**:543-558

[3] Yeh S, Tsai MY, Xu Q, Mu XM, Lardy H, Huang KE, et al. Generation and characterization of androgen receptor knockout (ARKO) mice: An in vivo model for the study of androgen functions in selective tissues. Proceedings of the National Academy of Sciences. 2002;**99**:13498-13503

[4] Cousins FL, Murray AA, Scanlon JP, Saunders PT. Hypoxyprobe reveals dynamic spatial and temporal changes in hypoxia in a mouse model of endometrial breakdown and repair. BMC Research Notes. 2016;**9**:30

[5] Cunha GR, Sinclair A, Ricke WA, Robboy SJ, Cao M, Baskin LS. Reproductive tract biology: Of mice and men. HHS Public Access. 2020;**110**:49-63

[6] Qureshi AS, Hussain M, Rehan S, Akbar Z, Rehman NU. Morphometric and angiogenic changes in the corpus luteum of nili-ravi buffalo (*Bubalus bubalis*) during estrous cycle. Pakistan Journal of Agricultural Sciences. 2015;**52**(3):795-800

[7] Lohmiller J, Swing SP. Reproduction and breeding. In: Suckow MA, Weisbroth SH, Franklin CL, editors. The Laboratory Rat. 2nd ed. Burlington, Vermont: Academic Press; 2006. pp. 147-164

[8] Drake AJ, van den Driesche S, Scott HM, Hutchison GR, Seckl JR, et al. Glucocorticoids amplify dibutyl phthalate induced disruption of testosterone production and male reproductive development. Endocrinology. 2009;**150**:5055-5064

[9] Takasu et al. Recovery from age-related infertility under environmental light-dark cycles adjusted to the intrinsic circadian period. Cell Reports. 2015;**12**:1407-1413

[10] Fata JE, Chaudhary V, Khokha R. Cellular turnover in the mammary gland is correlated with systemic levels of progesterone and not 17b-estradiol during the estrous cycle. Biology of Reproduction. 2001;**65**:680-688

[11] Goldman JM, Murr AS, Cooper RL. The rodent estrous cycle: Characterization of vaginal cytology and its utility in toxicological studies. Birth Defects Research B. 2007;**80**:84-97

[12] Baskin L, Shen J, Sinclair A, Cao M, Liu X, Liu G, et al. Development of the human penis and clitoris. Differentiation. 2018;**103**:74-85

[13] Overland M, Li Y, Cao M, Shen J, Yue X, Botta S, et al. Canalization of the vestibular plate in the absence of urethral fusion characterizes development of the human clitoris: The single zipper hypothesis. The Journal of Urology. 2016;**195**:1275-1283

[14] Hubscher CH, Brooks DL, Johnson JR. A quantitative method for assessing stages of the rat estrous cycle. Biotechnic & Histochemistry. 2005;**80**:79-87

[15] Elvis-Offiah UB, Bafor EE, Eze GI, Igbinumwen O, Viegelmann C, Edrada-Ebel R. In vivo investigation of female reproductive functions and parameters in nonpregnant mice models and mass spectrometric analysis of the methanol leaf extract of Emilia Coccinea (Sims) G Dons. Physiological Reports. 2016;**4**(23):e13047. DOI: 10.14814/phy2.13047

[16] Kooistra CM, Travlos G. Vaginal cytology of the laboratory rat and mouse: Review and criteria for the staging of the estrous cycle using stained vaginal smears. Toxicologic Pathology. 2015;**43**:776-793

[17] Byers SL, Wiles MV, Dunn SL, Taft RA. Mouse estrous cycle identification tool and images. PLoS One. 2012;**7**:1-5

[18] Grasso P, Rozhavskaya M, Reichert LE. In vivo effects of human follicle-stimulating hormone-related synthetic peptide hFSH-b- (90-95) on the mouse estrous cycle. Biology of Reproduction. 1998;**58**:821-825

[19] Bafor EE, Ukpebor F, Elvis-Offiah U, Uchendu A, Omoruyi O, Omogiade GU. Justicia flava leaves exert mild estrogenic activity in mouse models of uterotrophic and reproductive cycle investigations. Journal of Medicinal Food. 2019;**00**:1-14

[20] Morley-Fletcher S, Palanza P, Parolaro D, Vigano D, Laviola G. Intrauterine position has long-term influence on brain μ-opioid receptor density and behaviour in mice. Psychoneuroendocrinology. 2003;**28**:386-400

[21] Howdeshell KL, Wilson VS, Furr J, Lambright CR, Rider CV, Blystone CR, et al. A mixture of five phthalate esters inhibits fetal testicular testosterone production in the Sprague-Dawley Rat in a cumulative, dose-additive manner. Toxicological Sciences. 2008;**105**(1):153-165

[22] Caligioni CS. Assessing reproductive status/stages in mice. Current Protocols in Neuroscience. 2009;**48**(1). DOI: 10.1002/0471142301.nsa04is48

[23] Kent GC, Carr RK. Comparative Anatomy of the Vertebrates. 9th ed. New York: McGraw-Hill Companies; 2001

[24] Li S, Davis B. Evaluating rodent vaginal and uterine histology in toxicity studies. Birth Defects Research. Part B, Developmental and Reproductive Toxicology. 2007;**80**:246-252

[25] Van Der Lee S, Boot LM. Spontaneous pseudopregnancy in mice. Acta Physiologica et Pharmacologica Neerlandica. 1955;**4**:442-444

[26] Stockard CR, Papanicolaou CN. The existence of a typical oestrous cycle in the guinea-pig with a study of its histological and physiological changes. The American Journal of Anatomy. 1917;**22**:225-283

[27] Champlin AK, Darrold LD. Determining the stage of the estrous cycle in the mouse by the appearance of the vagina. Biology of Reproduction. 1973;**8**:491-494

[28] Elvis-Offiah UB, Bafor EE. Evaluation of the effects of oxytocin and diethylstilboesterol on mouse oestrous cycle using an Index. JMBR. 2014;**13**:5-16

[29] Organisation for the Economic Co-operation and Development (OECD). Part 5: Preparation, reading and reporting of vaginal smears. n.d. Available from: http://www.oecd.org/chemicalsafety/testing/40581357.pdf. [Accessed: April 1, 2014]

[30] Rottenfusser R. Proper alignment of the microscope. Methods in Cell Biology. 2013;**114**:43-67

Chapter 7

The Use of Astaxanthin as a Natural Antioxidant on Ovarian Damage

Abdulsamed Kükürt, Mahmut Karapehlivan and Volkan Gelen

Abstract

The ovaries are defined as the organs that secrete sex hormones and ensure the formation of the ovum in females. The proper functioning of the physiological functions of the ovaries is very important for the health of both the body and the female reproductive system. Reactive oxygen species are produced as byproducts of the normal physiological metabolism of the ovary. Antioxidants are among the factors that work to maintain the balance between the production and excretion of reactive oxygen species. Since the deterioration in the antioxidant system can cause pathological results, antioxidant supplementation is considered a possible strategy for the treatment of reproductive diseases by keeping oxidative stress under control. This chapter provides information about the use of astaxanthin as a natural antioxidant against ovarian damage.

Keywords: astaxanthin, *haematococcus pluvialis*, oxidative stress, antioxidant, ovarian damage

1. Introduction

The ovaries, which are the main reproductive organs of female mammals, consist of structures called follicles. These follicles contain granulosa cells in the early developmental stages and oocyte that can be translated by two somatic cell types called theca cells in the later stages of follicular development. These granulosa and theca cells together produce the sex steroid hormones estrogen and progesterone. At birth, an ovarian follicle reserve is established, which is generally regarded as a nonrenewable pool. It is noted that these limited number of follicles are required to support fertility throughout a female's lifetime through the production of a fertilizable gamete [1].

Reserve follicles that exist in the ovary after birth are activated by developmental stages called follicular waves throughout life. Follicle excretion occurs with the onset of ovulation cycles, especially with puberty. Therefore, a female continues her life with the number of oocytes present in her ovaries at birth. The number of these reserves, which exist with follicular waves, decreases over time and is depleted. In humans, this situation appears as menopause [2, 3].

Due to today's bad environmental conditions, uncontrolled use of pesticides, cheats in the food sector and various poisonings, there is a decrease in fertility rates or serious decreases in fertility in males and females. Infertility occurs and reproductive

IntechOpen

ability is disrupted, especially as the chemicals taken to impair the quality of the oocyte, prevent implantation, impair the quality of life of the sperm in the female genital tract after mating, cause early embryonal deaths, and directly or indirectly affect sexual activity [4].

It has been reported that physiologically low levels of reactive oxygen species (ROS) play an important role as an important regulator in various signal transduction pathways from folliculogenesis, oogenesis, embryogenesis, and pregnancy [5]. It has been stated that high levels of ROS, caused by increased production of oxidant species and/or decreased effectiveness of the antioxidant system, can lead to oxidative stress [6]. Nitric oxide is a mediator involved in vital functions such as the release of gonadotropins, steroidogenesis, folliculogenesis, ovulation, luteal development, luteolysis, and pregnancy. Thanks to the functions it has loaded in line with a dynamic order in the body, reproductive activities are fulfilled, while the opposite effect can be seen in excess. However, the fact that nitric oxide and nitric oxide synthases (eNOS, iNOS) are involved in the production of oocyte is an indication that it takes a role even in activities necessary for the continuation of life [7].

Excessive ROS production can occur in the organism due to many factors (exposure to chemicals, infectious agents, diseases, etc.). It has been suggested that the accumulation of high concentrations of ROS in the ovary causes detrimental effects on follicular function and plays an important role in the development of female reproductive diseases [8]. It has been suggested that oxidative stress in the ovaries causes granulosa cell apoptosis and follicular atresia in the follicles and damages oocytes [9]. Many studies have reported that granulosa cell apoptosis, one of the main causes of follicular atresia in mammals, is caused by oxidative stress [6, 10–12]. There are many defense mechanisms to prevent the formation of ROS so that it does not harm the organism. These mechanisms are often referred to as “antioxidant defense systems” or “antioxidants”. Antioxidants control the metabolism and free radical levels that occur in normal metabolic or pathological conditions and prevent or repair the damage that these radicals can cause [13–15].

It is reported that antioxidants are defense agents that play an important role in maintaining oxidative balance in the organism and protecting cells from the harmful effects of oxidative stress [6, 16, 17]. This chapter aimed to provide information about the use of antioxidants against experimentally induced oxidative ovarian damage.

2. Astaxanthin

Astaxanthin is a xanthophyll carotenoid found in various microorganisms and marine organisms [18]. Carotenoids can be synthesized naturally by cyanobacteria, algae, plants, some fungi, and some bacteria, but not by mammals. It has been noted that intake of carotenoids from food sources reduces the risk of many diseases such as breast, lung, ovary, colorectal, prostate cancer, and cardiovascular or eye diseases due to the antioxidant properties of carotenoids [19]. It has been reported that astaxanthin has stronger biological activity than other carotenoids [20].

Astaxanthin is obtained from seafood or *Haematococcus pluvialis*. *Haematococcus pluvialis* is a green microalgae that accumulates high astaxanthin content under stress conditions such as high salinity, nitrogen deficiency, high temperature, and light [21]. Astaxanthin produced from *Haematococcus pluvialis* is the main source for human consumption [22]. Astaxanthin is used as a pigment source in salmon, trout, and shrimp feeds [18]. It is stated that the consumption of astaxanthin, which is used as a dietary supplement in humans and animals, can prevent or reduce the risks of various disorders in humans and animals [23]. It is stated that the use of astaxanthin as a nutritional supplement is increasing rapidly in foods, feeds, nutraceuticals, and drugs [24].

Natural sources of astaxanthin are algae, moss, yeast, salmon, trout, krill, shrimp, and crayfish. Commercial astaxanthin is mainly produced by Phaffia yeast, *Haematococcus,* and chemical synthesis. *Haematococcus pluvialis* constitutes one of the best sources of natural astaxanthin [25]. It has been reported that shrimp, crab, and salmon can be preferred for dietary astaxanthin intake. It is suggested that 3.6 mg of astaxanthin supplementation per day may be beneficial for health [26].

Astaxanthin is a carotenoid containing carbon, hydrogen, and oxygen atoms in its structure (**Figure 1**). Consisting of two terminal rings linked by a polyene chain, this molecule has two asymmetric carbons located at the 3.3′ positions of the β-ionone ring with a hydroxyl (-OH) group at both ends. If the -OH group reacts with a fatty acid, a mono-ester is formed, and when both -OH groups react with fatty acids, a di-ester is formed as a result [18].

Astaxanthin can be found in various forms such as stereoisomer, geometric isomer, free and esterified [18]. Stereoisomers (3S, 3′S) and (3R 3′R) are the most abundant in nature. While *Haematococcus* biosynthesizes the (3S, 3′S)-isomer, yeast produces the *Xanthophyllomyces dendrorhous* (3R,3′R)-isomer [27]. It consists of synthetic astaxanthin (3S, 3′S) (3R, 3′S) and (3R, 3′R) isomers [28]. Astaxanthin has the molecular formula $C_{40}H_{52}O_4$ and its molar mass is 596.84 g/mol [18].

Astaxanthin contains conjugated double bond, -OH, and keto groups and has both lipophilic and hydrophilic properties [18]. The red color is due to the conjugated double bond in the middle of the compound. It is noted that due to the presence of such double bonds, they act as a strong antioxidant by donating electrons and reacting with free radicals to become a more stable product [23]. It has been reported that the ability to bind with the cell membrane from the inside out gives astaxanthin the ability to display better biological activity than other antioxidants [29, 30]. It is noted that oxidative molecules, which are reported to cause oxidative damage, can be inhibited by endogenous and exogenous antioxidants such as carotenoids, and astaxanthin is one of the antioxidant molecules that can inhibit oxidation [31].

Carotenoids are composed of a long-conjugated double-linked polyene chain that exerts antioxidant activity by quenching singlet oxygen and scavenger radicals to terminate chain reactions. It has been suggested that the biological benefits of carotenoids are due to their antioxidant properties resulting from their physical and chemical interaction with cell membranes and that astaxanthin has higher antioxidant activity compared to various carotenoids such as lutein, lycopene, α-carotene, and β-carotene [31, 32].

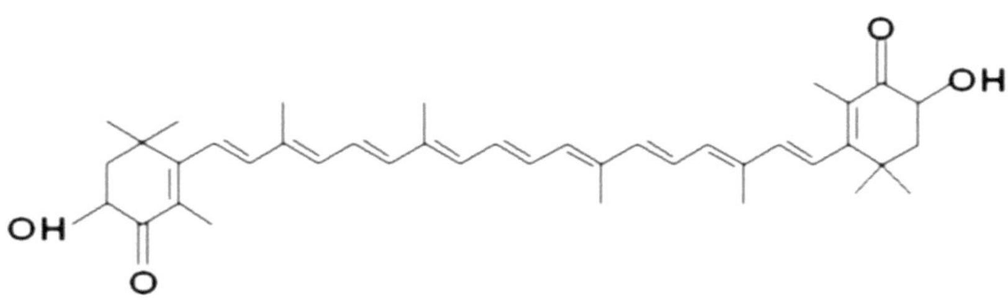

Figure 1.
Molecular structure of astaxanthin [18].

2.1 Possible effects of astaxanthin on ovaries

The ovarian follicle reserve created in fetal life is not renewed throughout the life of the creature. These limited number of reserve follicles are activated by developmental stages called follicular waves throughout life. Especially with the onset of ovulating cycles with puberty, follicle excretion occurs. Therefore, a female continues her life with the gradual decrease in the number of oocytes in her ovaries. Today, due to bad environmental conditions, uncontrolled use of pesticides, cheats in the food sector and various poisonings, there is a decrease in fertility rates or serious decreases in fertility in males and females. The chemicals taken especially impair the quality of the oocyte, prevent implantation, impair the quality of life of the sperm in the female genital tract after mating, cause early embryonal deaths, or affect sexual activity directly or indirectly, causing infertility and hindering reproductive ability [4, 33].

Physiologically low levels of ROS play a role as an important regulator of various signal transduction pathways in folliculogenesis, oogenesis, embryogenesis, and pregnancy [5]. High levels of ROS, caused by increased production of oxidant species and/or decreased effectiveness of the antioxidant system, lead to oxidative stress [14, 34–39]. Therefore, ovarian oxidative stress models will make important contributions to the understanding of these relationships, since the relationships between oxidative stress induced by ROS and the female reproductive system are not fully understood [40].

In the study in which experimental ovarian damage was created with 3-nitropropionic acid, the protective effect of astaxanthin against oxidative damage caused by 3-nitropropionic acid-induced ovarian toxicity was associated with its strong antioxidant effect. It was determined by the researchers that 3-nitropropionic acid injection caused a decrease in total antioxidant capacity levels and significant increases in total oxidant capacity and oxidative stress index levels in both ovaries and plasma. Also, while 3-nitropropionic acid caused an increase in sialic acid levels, this increase was suppressed by astaxanthin. In the study, it was determined that astaxanthin stopped the decrease in 3-nitropropionic acid-induced paraoxonase activity. It has been suggested that the use of astaxanthin may be beneficial in the prophylaxis and treatment of oxidative stress-related diseases, especially in infertility problems caused by ovarian degeneration [17].

In a study by Toktay et al. [41], they tried astaxanthin treatment against oxidative stress caused by ischemia-reperfusion in rat ovaries and achieved positive results. In the study, it was found that astaxanthin decreased lipid peroxidation and increased superoxide dismutase activity. In the same study, it was determined that astaxanthin decreased the increased caspase 3, IL-1 β, and IL-6 expressions. In another study, it was found that oxidative stress (total antioxidant status, total oxidant status, and oxidative stress index), apoptosis (caspase-3), and inflammation (c-reaktif protein, inducible nitric oxide synthase, granulocyte colony-stimulating factors) caused by methotrexate treatment in the urogenital tissue were improved with astaxanthin [42]. Ebrahimi et al. [43] reported that the administration of astaxanthin could reduce the oxidative stress factor H_2O_2 and apoptosis, while it increased the level of AKT protein expression.

A histopathological study revealed that the reduction in apico-basal height and cellular disruption in the uterine epithelium elicited by ovariectomy, signs of degeneration of the uterine glands, and inflammation in the stroma showed near-control improvement in astaxanthin-treated rats [44]. In an in vitro study, Kamada et al. [45] found that low concentrations of astaxanthin (0.1 to 10 nM) increased progesterone production in cultured bovine luteal cells, demonstrating the potential to improve corpus luteum function in cows. In ruminants, the oxidative stress index in the luteal phase where progesterone is high is higher than in the follicular phase. During the critical period of pregnancy, the high index of oxidative stress-induced progesterone causes embryonic death. Stress-inducing factors in high milk-yielding cows may affect the amount of progesterone synthesis by inhibiting luteal cell function due to excessive free radical production [46]. Abdel-Ghani et al. [47] showed that astaxanthin significantly increased the synthesis and secretion of estradiol in follicles and decreased the synthesis and secretion of progesterone. Li et al. [48] revealed that astaxanthin improves the development of follicles and oocytes by increasing the antioxidant capacity of follicles and oocytes and alleviating bisphenol A-induced oxidative stress during follicular development and oocyte maturation. Jia et al. [49] reported that astaxanthin treatment significantly reduced the production of reactive species in oocytes and improved the quality of oocytes. Xiu-Zhen et al. [50] showed that astaxanthin combined treatment considerably inhibited nuclear factor kappa B expression and translocation to the nucleus, thereby improving the astaxanthin-induced cytotoxic effect on the ovarian cystadenocarcinoma cell line.

3. Conclusion

The reproductive ability of the ovaries, which have an important role in female health, is impaired and infertility occurs due to many other problems that directly or indirectly affect sexual activity, such as bad environmental conditions, uncontrolled pesticide use, cheating in the food sector, and various poisonings. It is necessary to protect the health of the ovaries against the aforementioned negative factors for the prevention of infertility and therefore the continuation of the living species. For this purpose, the effects of the use of astaxanthin as a protective or therapeutic antioxidant agent against various agents that negatively affect ovarian health are discussed. As a result, when the studies were viewed, it was seen that astaxanthin can be used as a preventive and therapeutic in various ovarian damage cases due to its antioxidant, anti-inflammatory, antiapoptotic, and anticancer effects. In the light of all these data, we believe that the use of astaxanthin, a natural antioxidant agent, will be beneficial for the protection of the ovaries.

Author details

Abdulsamed Kükürt[1*], Mahmut Karapehlivan[2] and Volkan Gelen[3]

1 Faculty of Veterinary Medicine, Department of Biochemistry, Kafkas University, Kars, Türkiye

2 Faculty of Medicine, Department of Biochemistry, Kafkas University, Kars, Türkiye

3 Faculty of Veterinary Medicine, Department of Physiology, Kafkas University, Kars, Türkiye

*Address all correspondence to: samedkukurt@gmail.com

References

[1] Hirshfield AN. Development of follicles in the mammalian ovary. International Review of Cytology. 1991;**124**:43-101. DOI: 10.1016/S0074-7696(08)61524-7

[2] Cox E, Takov V. Embryology, ovarian follicle development. In: Treasure Island. Florida: StatPearls Publishing; 2022

[3] Desai N, Ludgin J, Sharma R, Anirudh RK, Agarwal A. Female and male gametogenesis. In: Falcone T, Hurd WW, editors. Clinical Reproductive Medicine and Surgery. New York: Springer; 2017. pp. 19-45. DOI: 10.1007/978-3-319-52210-4_2

[4] Sengupta P, Banerjee R. Environmental toxins: Alarming impacts of pesticides on male fertility. Human & Experimental Toxicology. 2014;**33**:1017-1039. DOI: 10.1177/0960327113515504

[5] Agarwal A, Gupta S, Sekhon L, Shah R. Redox considerations in female reproductive function and assisted reproduction: From molecular mechanisms to health implications. Antioxid Redox Signal. 2008;**10**:1375-1404. DOI: 10.1089/ars.2007.1964

[6] Ciani F, Cocchia N, D'Angelo D, Tafuri S. Influence of ROS on ovarian functions. In: Wu B, editor. New Discoveries in Embryology. London: IntechOpen; 2015. DOI: 10.5772/61003

[7] Kükürt A, Kuru M, Karapehlivan M. Nitrik oksit, nitrik oksit sentaz ve dişi üreme sistemindeki rolleri. In: Evereklioğlu C, editor. Saglik Bilimleri Alaninda Akademik Calismalar - II. Ankara: Gece Publishing; 2020. pp. 113-123

[8] Agarwal A, Gupta S, Sharma RK. Role of oxidative stress in female reproduction. Reproductive Biology and Endocrinology. 2005;**3**:28. DOI: 10.1186/1477-7827-3-28

[9] Jančar N, Kopitar AN, Ihan A, Klun IV, Bokal EV. Effect of apoptosis and reactive oxygen species production in human granulosa cells on oocyte fertilization and blastocyst development. Journal of Assisted Reproduction and Genetics. 2007;**24**:91-97. DOI: 10.1007/s10815-006-9103-8

[10] Murdoch WJ. Inhibition by oestradiol of oxidative stress-induced apoptosis in pig ovarian tissues. Journal of Reproduction and Fertility. 1998;**114**:127-130. DOI: 10.1530/jrf.0.1140127

[11] Zhang JQ, Xing BS, Zhu CC, Shen M, Yu FX, Liu HL. Protective effect of proanthocyanidin against oxidative ovarian damage induced by 3-nitropropionic acid in mice. Genetics and Molecular Research. 2015;**14**:2484-2494. DOI: 10.4238/2015.March.30.6

[12] Li B, Weng Q, Liu Z, Shen M, Zhang J, Wu W, et al. Selection of antioxidants against ovarian oxidative stress in mouse model. Journal of Biochemical and Molecular Toxicology. 2017;**31**:e21997. DOI: 10.1002/jbt.21997

[13] Kükürt A, Kuru M, Başer ÖF, Karapehlivan M. Kisspeptin: Role in female infertility. In: Marsh C, editor. Reproductive Hormones. London: IntechOpen; 2021. pp. 174-186. DOI: 10.5772/intechopen.94925

[14] Gelen V, Kükürt A, Şengül E, Başer ÖF, Karapehlivan M. Can polyphenols be used as anti-inflammatory agents against Covid-19 (SARS-CoV-2)-induced inflammation? In: Badria FA, editor. Phenolic Compounds - Chemistry,

Synthesis, Diversity, Non-Conventional Industrial, Pharmaceutical and Therapeutic Applications. London: IntechOpen; 2022. pp. 341-361. DOI: 10.5772/intechopen.98684

[15] Kükürt A, Gelen V, Başer ÖF, Deveci HA, Karapehlivan M. Thiols: Role in oxidative stress-related disorders. In: Atukeren P, editor. Accent. Lipid Peroxidation. London: IntechOpen; 2021. pp. 27-47. DOI: 10.5772/intechopen.96682

[16] Davies KJ. Oxidative stress: The paradox of aerobic life. Biochem Soc Symp. 1995. p. 61. DOI: 10.1042/bss0610001

[17] Kükürt A, Karapehlivan M. Protective effect of astaxanthin on experimental ovarian damage in rats. Journal of Biochemical and Molecular Toxicology. 2022;**36**:e22966. DOI: 10.1002/jbt.22966

[18] Higuera-Ciapara I, Félix-Valenzuela L, Goycoolea FM. Astaxanthin: A review of its chemistry and applications. Critical Reviews in Food Science and Nutrition. 2006;**46**:185-196. DOI: 10.1080/10408690590957188

[19] Merhan O. The biochemistry and antioxidant properties of carotenoids. In: Cvetkovic DJ, Nikolic GS, editors. Carotenoids. London: IntechOpen; 2017. DOI: 10.5772/67592

[20] Pashkow FJ, Watumull DG, Campbell CL. Astaxanthin: A novel potential treatment for oxidative stress and inflammation in cardiovascular disease. The American Journal of Cardiology. 2008;**101**:S58-S68. DOI: 10.1016/j.amjcard.2008.02.010

[21] Ravi S, Ambati RR, Sandesh BK, Chandrappa D, Narayanan A, Chauhan VS, et al. Influence of different culture conditions on yield of biomass and value added products in microalgae. Dynamic Biochemistry, Process Biotechnology and Molecular Biology. 2012;**6**:77-85

[22] Kidd P. Astaxanthin, cell membrane nutrient with diverse clinical benefits and anti-aging potential. Alternative Medicine Review. 2011;**16**:355-364

[23] Guerin M, Huntley ME, Olaizola M. Haematococcus astaxanthin: Applications for human health and nutrition. Trends in Biotechnology. 2003;**21**:210-216. DOI: 10.1016/S0167-7799(03)00078-7

[24] Ambati R, Phang S-M, Ravi S, Aswathanarayana R. Astaxanthin: Sources, extraction, stability, biological activities and its commercial applications—A review. Marine Drugs. 2014;**12**:128-152. DOI: 10.3390/md12010128

[25] Ranga Rao A, Raghunath Reddy RL, Baskaran V, Sarada R, Ravishankar GA. Characterization of microalgal carotenoids by mass spectrometry and their bioavailability and antioxidant properties elucidated in rat model. Journal of Agricultural and Food Chemistry. 2010;**58**:8553-8559. DOI: 10.1021/jf101187k

[26] Iwamoto T, Hosoda K, Hirano R, Kurata H, Matsumoto A, Miki W, et al. Inhibition of low-density lipoprotein oxidation by astaxanthin. Journal of Atherosclerosis and Thrombosis. 2000;**7**:216-222. DOI: 10.5551/jat1994.7.216

[27] Hussein G, Sankawa U, Goto H, Matsumoto K, Watanabe H. Astaxanthin, a carotenoid with potential in human health and nutrition. Journal of Natural Products. 2006;**69**:443-449. DOI: 10.1021/np050354+

[28] Foss P, Renstrøm B, Liaaen-Jensen S. Natural occurrence of enantiomeric and Meso astaxanthin 7∗-crustaceans including zooplankton. Comparative

Biochemistry and Physiology Part B: Comparative Biochemistry. 1987;**86**:313-314. DOI: 10.1016/0305-0491(87)90298-7

[29] Yuan J-P, Peng J, Yin K, Wang J-H. Potential health-promoting effects of astaxanthin: A high-value carotenoid mostly from microalgae. Molecular Nutrition & Food Research. 2011;**55**:150-165. DOI: 10.1002/mnfr.201000414

[30] Yamashita E. Astaxanthin as a medical food. Functional Foods in Health and Disease. 2013;**3**:254. DOI: 10.31989/ffhd.v3i7.49

[31] Naguib YMA. Antioxidant activities of astaxanthin and related carotenoids. Journal of Agricultural and Food Chemistry. 2000;**48**:1150-1154. DOI: 10.1021/jf991106k

[32] Merhan O, Özcan A, Atakişi E, Öğün M, Kükürt A. The effect of β-carotene on acute phase response in diethylnitrosamine given rabbits. Kafkas Univ Vet Fak Derg. 2016;**22**:533-537. DOI: 10.9775/kvfd.2016.14995

[33] Petrelli G, Mantovani A. Environmental risk factors and male fertility and reproduction. Contraception. 2002;**65**:297-300. DOI: 10.1016/S0010-7824(02)00298-6

[34] Gelen V, Şengül E, Yıldırım S, Senturk E, Tekin S, Kükürt A. The protective effects of hesperidin and curcumin on 5-fluorouracil–induced nephrotoxicity in mice. Environmental Science and Pollution Research. 2021;**34**:47046-47055. DOI: 10.1007/s11356-021-13969-5

[35] Gelen V, Kükürt A, Şengül E. Role of the renin-angiotensin-aldosterone system in various disease processes: An overview. In: McFarlane SI, editor. Renin-Angiotensin Aldosterone System. London: IntechOpen; 2021. pp. 55-78. DOI: 10.5772/intechopen.97354

[36] Kara A, Gedikli S, Sengul E, Gelen V, Ozkanlar S. Oxidative stress and autophagy. In: Ahmad R, editor. Free Radicals Disease. Rijeka: IntechOpen; 2016. pp. 69-86. DOI: 10.5772/64569

[37] Gelen V, Şengül E, Kükürt A. An overview of effects on reproductive physiology of melatonin. In: Gelen V, Şengül E, Kükürt A, editors. Melatonin - Recent Updates [Working Title]. London: IntechOpen; 2022. DOI: 10.5772/intechopen.108101

[38] Deveci HA, Nur G, Deveci A, Kaya I, Kaya MM, Kükürt A, et al. An overview of the biochemical and histopathological effects of insecticides. In: Ranz RER, editor. Insecticides - Impact and Benefits of Its Use for Humanity. London: IntechOpen; 2021. DOI: 10.5772/intechopen.100401

[39] Gelen V, Kükürt A, Şengül E, Deveci HA. Leptin and its role in oxidative stress and apoptosis: An overview. In: Rao V, Rao L, editors. Role of Obesity in Human Health and Disease. London: IntechOpen; 2021. pp. 143-163. DOI: 10.5772/intechopen.101237

[40] Zhang J-Q, Shen M, Zhu C-C, Yu F-X, Liu Z-Q, Ally N, et al. 3-Nitropropionic acid induces ovarian oxidative stress and impairs follicle in mouse. PLoS One. 2014;**9**:e86589. DOI: 10.1371/journal.pone.0086589

[41] Toktay E, Tastan TB, Gurbuz MA, Erbas E, Demir O, Ugan RA, et al. Potential protective effect of astaxanthin on ovary ischemia-reperfusion injury. Iranian Journal of Basic Medical Sciences. 2022;**25**:173-178. DOI: 10.22038/IJBMS.2022.61289.13559

[42] Gunyeli I, Saygin M, Ozmen O. Methotrexate-induced toxic effects and the ameliorating effects of astaxanthin on genitourinary tissues in a female rat model. Archives of Gynecology

and Obstetrics. 2021;**304**:985-997. DOI: 10.1007/s00404-021-06000-2

[43] Ebrahimi F, Rostami S, Nekoonam S, Rashidi Z, Sobhani A, Amidi F. The effect of astaxanthin and metformin on oxidative stress in granulosa cells of BALB C mouse model of polycystic ovary syndrome. Reproductive Sciences. 2021;**28**:2807-2815. DOI: 10.1007/s43032-021-00577-4

[44] Gürler EB, Kaya ÖT. Overektomi Uygulanan Sıçanlarda Uterus Dokuları Üzerinde Astaksantinin Etkisi: Histopatolojik Çalışma. Genel Tıp Derg. 2021;**31**:40-44

[45] Kamada H, Akagi S, Watanabe S. Astaxanthin increases progesterone production in cultured bovine luteal cells. Journal of Veterinary Medical Science. 2017;**79**:1103-1109. DOI: 10.1292/jvms.17-0044

[46] Kuru M, Kükürt A, Oral H, Öğün M. Clinical use of progesterone and its relation to oxidative stress in ruminants. In: Drevenšek G, editor. Sex Horm. Neurodegener. Process. Dis. Rijeka, London, UK: IntechOpen; 2018. pp. 303-327. DOI: 10.5772/intechopen.73311

[47] Abdel-Ghani MA, Yanagawa Y, Balboula AZ, Sakaguchi K, Kanno C, Katagiri S, et al. Astaxanthin improves the developmental competence of in vitro-grown oocytes and modifies the steroidogenesis of granulosa cells derived from bovine early antral follicles. Reproduction Fertility and Development. 2019;**31**:272. DOI: 10.1071/RD17527

[48] Li Y, Dong Z, Liu S, Gao F, Zhang J, Peng Z, et al. Astaxanthin improves the development of the follicles and oocytes through alleviating oxidative stress induced by BPA in cultured follicles. Scientific Reports. 2022;**12**:7853. DOI: 10.1038/s41598-022-11566-1

[49] Jia B-Y, Xiang D-C, Shao Q-Y, Zhang B, Liu S-N, Hong Q-H, et al. Inhibitory effects of astaxanthin on postovulatory porcine oocyte aging in vitro. Scientific Reports. 2020;**10**:20217. DOI: 10.1038/s41598-020-77359-6

[50] Su X-Z, Chen R, Wang C-B, Ouyang X-L, Jiang Y, Zhu M-Y. Astaxanthin combine with human serum albumin to abrogate cell proliferation, migration, and drug-resistant in human ovarian carcinoma SKOV3 cells. Anti-Cancer Agents in Medicinal Chemistry. 2019;**19**:792-801. DOI: 10.2174/1871520619666190225123003

Section 3

Aquatic Animal Health Research

Chapter 8

Erythrocytes and Hemoglobin of Fish: Potential Indicators of Ecological Biomonitoring

Atanas Arnaudov and Dessislava Arnaudova

Abstract

Anthropogenic pollution of the freshwater basins is a serious environmental problem. This has necessitated the search for different approaches to the detection of different pollutants in water bodies. Many authors point out that the hematological parameters of freshwater fish are sensitive to the action of various pollutants in freshwater basins. This chapter summarizes the results of studies on the effects of current water pollutants (heavy metals, organic matter, etc.) on erythrocytes and hemoglobin in fish. An analysis of the possibility of the use of erythrocyte damage and the change in the hemoglobin content of the tested animals for the purposes of ecological biomonitoring of freshwater pollution will be made.

Keywords: anemia, biomonitoring, ecotoxicology, erythrocyte abnormalities, teleost, water pollution

1. Introduction

The state of the environment is signaled by a group of different biological species known as bioindicators. They are responsible for demonstrating the impact of different types of pollutants. The selection of a specific biological species as an indicator should be done considering its sensitivity to various changes in the environment [1]. Fishes are valuable species as bioindicators for the pollution of water bodies. A very large number and essentially different methods can be applied to them, which allow assessment of the severity of toxic effects by determining the accumulation of toxic substances in the tissues, by using histological and hematological approaches. Thus, bioindication using fish represents a good tool for biomonitoring, regarding both pollution and river engineering aspects, e.g., river restoration and management [2].

In this chapter, our and other authors' summarized data on the possibilities of using the erythrocyte indicators of teleost fishes for the purposes of biomonitoring will be presented.

IntechOpen

2. Erythrocytes and hemoglobin in teleost in the norm and under toxic effects

2.1 Erythrocytes and hemoglobin in teleost in the norm

The erythrocytes of teleost fishes have a similar morphology to the erythrocytes of other non-mammalian vertebrates. They are nucleated cells with an elliptical to oval shape. Their cytoplasm is eosinophilic, and the nucleus is centrally located, deeply basophilic, with an oval to elliptical shape. Erythrocyte sizes range from 102 to 800 fl [3, 4]. Moderate anisocytosis and polychromasia are normal in teleost species.

Their life span is 13–500 days. The number of erythrocytes in the peripheral blood depends on many factors—fish activity, water temperature, and dissolved oxygen concentration, as well as other environmental factors and shows significant seasonal variability. Furthermore, it depends on age, sex, nutritional and reproductive status, and may differ between populations of the same species. It typically ranges from $0.5–1.5 \times 10^6/mm^3$ in less active species to $3.0–4.2 \times 10^6/mm^3$ in more active species. Antarctic icefishes, adapted to cold and well-oxygenated water, do not have erythrocytes.

The main erythropoietic organ in teleost is the head kidney. Erythropoiesis is similar to that of other vertebrates and involves the same precursors. Characteristically, in teleost fishes, the barrier between the hematopoietic tissue and the circulatory system is weak, and therefore in the circulating blood, many immature red blood cells are found, often constituting more than 10% of all erythrocytes. Immature erythrocytes are round rather than oval in shape, their cytoplasm is blue-stained, and their nucleus is larger and heterochromatic.

As in other vertebrates, fish erythrocytes contain tetrameric hemoglobins, but with different oxygen affinities. It is lower in species living in well-oxygenated water than in those exposed to hypoxia. Several hemoglobin isoforms with different oxygen affinities are often present in the blood of fish, which is considered an adaptation to variable oxygen concentration in the water. Fish erythrocytes are sensitive to environmental pollution, and their morphological assessment can be used as a bioindicator of toxicity [3].

2.2 Hematological disorders in teleost as a biomarker for water pollution

Hematologic studies in fish have been performed for more than 70 years now. Recently, they have gained great importance because they are an effective and sensitive indicator for evaluating physiological and pathological changes caused by natural or anthropogenic pollution of water sources. Hematological indicators are therefore considered an important tool to identify the functional state of the body in response to various stressors [5]. However, for the correct interpretation of the obtained results, it is necessary to consider a set of variables, such as reproductive cycle, age, sex, feeding behavior, stress, nutritional status, and water quality, as well as the habitat of the species, since poikilothermic animals are under the impact of environmental changes [6].

Hematological disorders in boteleost include anemia, polycythemia, abnormal morphology, and cytoplasmic and nuclear inclusions [4], and according to Witeska [3], they also include changes in the size and color of erythrocytes.

Anemia is well described in teleost. It is defined as a decrease in hemoglobin concentration below the reference level of an established threshold for a population of healthy organisms [7]. In teleost it is extremely difficult to establish reference values for hematological parameters, due to their strong variation caused by their poikilothermism and high sensitivity to the action of various factors (age, sex, water quality, photoperiod, season, diet, etc.). For example, hematocrit values strongly depend on the level of biological activity of the fish. Thus, actively swimming species such as tuna and other pelagic species generally have much higher hematocrit values than bottom-dwelling fish such as flatfish. Therefore, hematological parameters are very relative, and there is no clear definition of normal and abnormal values [8]. Therefore, anemia in fish is usually recognized by a significant reduction in red blood parameters compared with the values obtained for a reference group of animals not exposed to the specific damaging factor. According to Clauss et al. [4], hematocrit values (PCV) below 20% are indicative of anemia. The hematological parameters that are affected when anemia occurs in fish are mainly: red blood cell count (RBC), hemoglobin concentration (Hb), hematocrit, mean corpuscular volume (MCV), mean corpuscular hemoglobin content (MCH), and mean corpuscular hemoglobin concentration (MCHC). Examination of these indicators (along with WBC values) is recommended for routine monitoring of fish health status in fish farms [9].

Anemia in teleost fishes occurs under both natural and aquaculture conditions and can be caused by various effects, including the toxic effect of a number of pollutants in water bodies (nitrates, pesticides, heavy metal ions, cyanobacterial toxins, etc.) [3].

Depending on the causes of anemia, it can be hemorrhagic, hemolytic, or hypoplastic. Depending on the manifestations, the different types of anemia in fish are divided into microcytic, normocytic, and macrocytic (depending on the size of the erythrocytes), as well as hypochromic or normochromic (depending on the hemoglobin concentration) [4].

2.3 Hematological disorders of fish under toxic effects

2.3.1 Hematological disorders caused by the action of nitrites

Toxic concentrations of nitrites in fish breeding ponds can occur in intensive aquaculture systems as a consequence of high stocking density and feeding intensity. In natural water bodies, elevated nitrite levels usually result from sewage pollution. Prolonged exposure to nitrite induces oxidative stress in fish [10]. According to Witeska, nitrite intoxication can result in anemia, followed by oxidation of hemoglobin to methemoglobin [3]. Da Costa et al. [11] reported methemoglobinemia in *Colossoma macropomum*, caused by nitrite intoxication, accompanied by hemolytic anemia due to reduced erythrocyte life span. Erythrocyte hemolysis with prolonged exposure to nitrites results from a high expenditure of cellular energy to reduce methemoglobin, which shortens the average life span of red blood cells [10]. There is much evidence to show that the symptoms of anemia caused by nitrites can be different, which depends both on the severity of intoxication and on the biological species of the fish. Witeska [3] reported that in different types of fish, there can be a decrease in different parameters. Thus, in *Dicentricus labrax,* only the hemoglobin content tends to decrease, but in other species decrease is observed also in RBC and/or hematocrit, and in *Colossoma macropotum* and *Sander vitreus,* increase is even observed of

MCHC (probably as a compensatory reaction to the impaired oxygen transport from the blood). According to Zhelev et al. [12], elevated nitrate levels in a natural water basin (Sazliyka River, Bulgaria) induce erythrocytosis and hyperchromia in adult *Carassius gibelio* females.

Data on the effect of nitrate pollution of water bodies on the morphology of erythrocytes of fish are scarce.

2.3.2 Hematological disorders caused by the action of metals and microelements

The impact of toxic concentrations of metal ions in water bodies causes morpho-functional changes in erythrocytes, which can result in various negative effects: direct damage to erythrocyte cells, reduction of their life span, acceleration of hemolysis or inhibition of erythropoiesis.

There is a large number of publications on this subject in the literature, and in most cases the authors describe and explain the mechanisms of action of each individual heavy metal toxicant. According to Fedeli et al. [13], copper induces oxidative damage to erythrocytes and increases their susceptibility to hemolysis. Our studies confirm this, showing that the hematocrit of *C. gibelio* is reliably reduced even by the action of copper at concentrations lower than the threshold limit values (TLVs) for freshwater bodies (0.1 mg/l), but by the action of high concentrations (2.0 mg/l), its values are comparable to those of the controls. In our opinion, this is due to a compensatory increase in erythropoiesis, as a result of which young erythrocytes with insufficient hemoglobin content are found in the peripheral blood of the fish. Enhanced erythropoiesis under the action of high concentrations of copper was indirectly proven by histological examination of the spleen of *C. gibelio* [14]. Unlike the control group, in fish exposed to 2.0 mg/l copper sulfate, no presence of hemosiderin was detected in the spleen. This is an indication of mobilization of iron reserve in fish organisms. The type of anemia was different under the influence of different concentrations of copper sulfate: under the influence of concentrations of 0.1 and 2.0 mg/l, it was microcytic and hypochromic, under the influence of a concentration of 0.5 mg/l, it was microcytic and normochromic, and under the influence of a concentration of 1.0 mg/l, normocytic and normochromic.

Som et al. [15] reported a decrease in the amount of erythropoietic precursors in the head kidney of *Labeo rohita* associated with the level of copper intoxication. Cadmium, like copper, damages hematopoietic precursors in the kidney of *Ictalurus nebulosus* [16]. According to Kondera and Witeska [17], this may be due to an increase in apoptosis in precursor cells in copper or cadmium intoxication.

Results of our study [18] allow indicating some features related to changes in the sizes of erythrocytes and their nuclei under the influence of different concentrations of copper in water. Under the influence of low concentrations of copper (even below TLV), a decrease in the size of the cells and of their nuclei is identified. However, under the influence of higher concentrations of copper, an increase in the size of the cells is caused, which can be explained by the activation of compensatory processes.

The bases of Prise-Jones curves gave the following results:

- At the big diameter of erythrocytes, anisocytosis in concentrations of 0.1 and 1.0 mg/l was found.

- At the small diameter of erythrocytes, there is a widening of the curves bases, especially well expressed in 1.0 mg/l concentration.

- At the big diameter of the nuclei, there was a tendency of decreasing anisocytosis.
- At the small diameter of the nuclei, the fluctuations are near to the values of the controls.

A conclusion can be made that copper, even in concentrations below TLV for waters, causes atrophic changes in the erythrocytes of *C. gibelio*. This fact can be used for the purposes of ecological biomonitoring of copper contamination of water bodies.

According to Akahori et al. [19] and Gabryelak et al. [20], zinc induced hemolytic anemia in fish, which resulted from its adverse effect on the lipid layer of the erythrocyte membrane. In our studies, a negative effect of the action of different concentrations of zinc on different hematological parameters of *C. gibelio* was found. Changes were found in RBC, erythrocyte morphology, and size, Hb, PCV, MCV, MCH, and MCHC. From the analysis of the obtained results, it can be concluded that zinc causes hypochromic anemia even in low concentrations (below TLV). A trend of transition from microcytic to macrocytic type of anemia was observed with increasing zinc concentration. Witeska and Koś命ciuk [21] reported that hematocrit and frequency of abnormal erythrocytes in Common carp increased after a 3-hour exposure to 20 mg/dm^{-3} zinc (ZnO).

The changes in the shape (poikilocytosis) and in the sizes of erythrocytes were also different, under the action of the different concentrations of zinc. The beginning of the processes of karyopyknosis, hypertrophy and anisocytosis were detected [22–24]. Similar to the effect of copper, compensatory changes in erythrocyte size and erythrocyte indices were observed here as zinc concentration increased. In this case, similar to the effect of copper, an absence of hemosiderin was found in the spleen of fish subjected to the action of 2.0 mg/l zinc, which is an indication that a similar process of mobilization of the body's iron reserves is taking place.

Lead reduces the activity of ALA-D (a key enzyme involved in heme synthesis) [25, 26]. In our studies, we found that carp lead caused erythrocyte deformations with a clear upward trend proportional to increase in concentration [27]. After short-term exposure (96 h LC50), lead caused increase in frequency of morphological anomalies in carp erythrocytes over the entire experimental period. Cromatin condensation at the nucleus border and nuclear malformation were the most common anomalies. No complete recovery took place until the end of the experiment [28].

The effect of other metal pollutants in water (nickel, mercury, chromium, selenium, etc.) has been less studied. In our studies, it was found that nickel causes erythrocyte changes in carp, including with concentrations far below TLV [29]. Its main effect is damage to the cell membrane (which causes the appearance of poikilocytosis) and changes in the shape of cell nuclei. Under the influence of concentrations above TLV, necrotic changes occur in the nuclei (karyopyknosis). The established erythrocyte changes may be explained by the finding of De Luca et al. [30] that nickel affects cellular metabolism, causing an enhancement of oxidative stress in erythrocytes. In *Cirrhinus mrigala*, nickel causes significant decrease of RBC, Hb, and PCV [31]. According to Moosavi et al. [32], hematological and biochemical parameters can be used as an indicator of nickel-related stress in fish on exposure to elevated nickel status.

In general, it can be summarized that metal pollutants in water bodies cause a decrease in the values of hematological parameters of fish—most often (Hb, RBC, and PCV, and in some cases also MCV, MCH, and MCHC), but for some metals, there may be an increase in MCV (under the influence of copper and chromium) or in MCH under the influence of cadmium [3].

In natural conditions, hematological disorders can be caused by the action of mixtures of metal pollutants, and their effect on fish is the result of the combination of mechanisms of action of the contained metal pollutants in water bodies [33].

In 2007–2008, we conducted a study of hematological parameters of three species of freshwater fish—bleak (*Alburnus alburnus* L.), common rudd (*Scardinus erythrophtalmus* L.), and European perch (redfin perch) (*Perca fluviatilis* L.), inhabiting Studen Kladenets Dam (Arda River area, Bulgaria) [34]. Elevated levels of manganese and lead have been found in the waters of the dam. Anemic changes were found in the blood of the three species in both the summer and winter seasons. Each species, however, developed a different type of anemia—macrocytic and hyperchromic in bleak, hypochromic type in common rudd, and normochromic anemia, which developed into microcytic normochromic anemia in winter in redfin perch. Morphological examination of the erythrocytes of all three species of freshwater fish demonstrated a wide range of erythrocyte changes, as well as a large number of "amitotic" erythrocytes in the peripheral blood of common rudd and redfin perch. These changes showed interspecies differences. Later Omar et al. [35] found that high concentrations of heavy metal mixtures (Cu^{2+}, Zn^{2+}, Pb^{2+}, Fe^{2+} and Mn^{2+}) have a potential genotoxic effect on erythrocytes, in studies of cultured and wild Nile tilapia, *Oreochromis niloticus* and mullet *Mugil cephalus*, inhabiting a water body, contaminated with agricultural wastewater and domestic untreated water discharges (Lake Qaroun, Egypt). It has been shown that the genotoxic effect (measured by a micronucleus test) depends proportionally on the type and concentration of pollutants in the water body. In addition to micronuclei, other nuclear and cellular abnormalities have been reported in fish erythrocytes—lobular, vesicular, binucleate, dentate, budded, vacuolated and other deformed nuclei, karyolysis, nuclear retraction, as well as microcytes and vacuolated cytoplasm. Degradation of the studied aquatic habitats reveals species-specific effects.

In 2014/2015, a study of the cytometric characteristics of the erythrocytes of *C. gibelio* Bloch, 1782, and *Rutilus rutilus* (Linnaeus, 1758), inhabiting the Zaporizhya Reservoir (Ukraine), was conducted [36]. The species characteristic of accumulation of heavy metals in the body of carp fish was also investigated. It was established that young specimens of *C. gibelio* and *R. rutilus* accumulate essential elements, especially zinc, to a greater extent than adults. The level of intensity of occurrence of erythropoiesis was higher in young fish of both species. Specific features of the cytometric characteristics of fish erythrocytes were identified: the relative amount of mature red blood cells predominated in *R. rutilus*, and the area of mature red blood cells was significantly higher in *C. gibelio*. In addition, a significantly higher percentage of polychromatophilic normoblasts was found among the immature forms of red blood cells in juvenile *R. rutilus*.

According to Zhelev et al. [12], elevated levels of heavy metals in a natural water basin (Topolnitsa River, Bulgaria) induce erythrocytosis and microcytic hypochromic anemia in adult female *C. gibelio*.

2.3.3 Hematological disorders caused by the action of pesticides

Various pesticides used in agriculture and draining into water bodies have also been reported as agents causing various hematological disorders [3, 37, 38]. According to Mikula et al. [39], the pesticide alachlor in subchronic doses induced pathological changes in hematopoietic organs of carps (*Cyprinus carpio* L.) As a result, all hematological parameters were lower compared with the control group fish, except for PCV. Dogan and Can [40] suggested that dimethoate probably also has a damaging effect on fish erythropoietic tissue. In *Oncorhynchus mykiss*, in sublethal concentrations this pesticide caused a significant decrease in RBC, Hb, PCV, MCV, and MCH, indicating the occurrence of microcytic hypochromic anemia.

As reported by Ghaffar et al. [41], Fipronil causes a decrease of RBC, Hb, and PCV. It is assumed that the decrease of Hb may be due to its oxidation to methemoglobin, poorer gas exchange, and damage caused by free radicals. The authors assume that anemic changes are a marker of the weak role of hematopoietic tissues, inappropriate osmoregulatory mechanisms, and increased damage of red blood cells in hematopoietic organs. In another case, in *L. rohita*, exposure to Fipronil for 9 days at a dose of 0.03–0.15 mg/L showed various nuclear changes in addition to RBC reduction in erythrocytes.

According to Tahir et al., [37] a large number of pesticides (cypermethrin, triazophos, butachlor, DDT, BHC, aldrin, dieldrin, chlordane, permethrin, cypermethrin, karate, delmethrin sulfane, endosulfan, etc.) cause anemic changes in various teleost, with *L. rohita* being a suitable model for studying the damaging effects of pesticides.

In some cases, the hematopoietic system of fish has the ability to compensate for the action of pesticides. This was found by Hii et al. [42], who reported that endosulfan induced in *Monopterus albus* a short-term increase of RBC, Hb, and PCV, which is followed by a significant decrease in the values of these indicators, due to the damaging effect of the pesticide on the erythrocyte membrane.

Some pesticides have also been found to cause DNA damage in fish erythrocytes [37], in addition to affecting the main hematological parameters (RBC, Hb, and PCV, etc.). Thus, naphthalene-2-sulphonate caused genotoxic effects on *Channa punctatus*, which was detected by comet assay and micronucleus assay. A mixture of endosulfan and Chlorpyrifos can also induce DNA damage in the erythrocytes of *O. niloticus*, which was found by Ambreen and Javed [43] by comet assay.

The data cited above show that the study of erythrocyte indicators in natural and laboratory conditions is a good opportunity to establish the harmful effect of newly synthesized pesticides, which would help to determine their harmful effects, and based on these studies, more less toxic and environmentally friendly chemicals could be used [37].

2.3.4 Hematological disorders caused by the action of cyanobacterial toxins

Cyanobacteria inhabit both freshwater and saltwater bodies throughout the world. In case of excessive growth leading to eutrophication, they can produce specific toxins (cyanotoxins) in quantities causing toxicity, including in humans. Cyanotoxins are cyclic peptides and alkaloids. Cyclic peptides include microcystins and nodularins. Alkaloids include anatoxin-a, anatoxin-a(S), cylindrospermopsin, saxitoxins (STXs), aplisiatoxins, and lingbiatoxin [44]. The effects of microcystin have been best studied on teleost. According to Witeska [3], there are species differences in the sensitivity of fish to the action of this toxin. According to Zhang et al. [45], microcystin in high doses caused in *Carassius auratus* a significant decrease of RBC, Hb, and PCV in the high-dose group and Hb, while the erythrocyte sedimentation rate (ESR) was significantly increased, indicating the occurrence of normocytic anemia. No significant deviations were found in MCV, MCH, and MCHC. Under the action of low doses of the toxin, hematological disorders are reversible. According to the authors, such hematological disorders are due to impairment of erythropoiesis. In the same species, Zhou et al. [46] found that microcystin significantly increased lipid peroxidation as well as the activity of antioxidant enzymes. These changes cause erythrocyte malformation, cell membrane damage that increases hemolysis, i.e., there is another mechanism causing anemia (oxidative damage to erythrocytes).

Based on data, provided by Navratil et al. [47], microcystin induces in *Cyprinus caprio* hemorrhagic anemia, which is a consequence of extensive hemorrhages in the skin, hepatopancreas, and eyes. On the other hand, however, there are data that microcystin formed both by natural eutrophication and by cyanobacterial isolates does not cause any anemic changes in *Cyprinus caprio* (according to Witeska [3]).

3. Conclusion

Teleost fishes possess a high compensatory potential for improving oxygen transport under the influence of adverse environmental factors [48]. It includes synthesis of erythrocytes and hemoglobin, amitotic division of erythrocytes, release of erythrocytes from blood depots (spleen and main kidney), as well as activation of hematopoiesis.

A low-cost response to oxygen deficiency is realized by increasing the MCV. The increase in cell volume, together with the increase in erythrocyte pH, improves oxygen transport under hypoxic conditions [3]. They result from adrenergic activation of Na^+/proton exchange across the erythrocyte membrane [49]. Knowledge, on the one hand, of anemic and genotoxic effects of aquatic pollutants, and on the other hand, of adaptive-compensatory responses to the action of aquatic toxicants, is a good basis for using a large set of freshwater bony fish for ecological biomonitoring purposes.

Acknowledgement

This chapter is published with support of NPD-Plovdiv University "Paisii Hilendarski" under Project № PP22-BF-005.

Conflict of interest

The authors declare no conflict of interest.

Author details

Atanas Arnaudov* and Dessislava Arnaudova
Plovdiv University "P. Hilendarski", Plovdiv, Bulgaria

*Address all correspondence to: arny87@abv.bg

References

[1] Asif N, Malik M, Chaudhry FN. A review of on environmental pollution bioindicators. Pollution. 2018;**4**(1):111-118. DOI: 10.22059/poll.2017.237440.296

[2] Chovanec A, Hofer R, Schiemer F. Fish as bioindicators. Bioindicators & Biomonitors. In: Trace Metals and Other Contaminants in the Environment. Oxford, UK: Elsevier; 2003. pp. 639-676

[3] Witeska M. Anemia in teleost fishes. Bulletin of the European Association of Fish Pathologist. 2008;**35**(4):148-160

[4] Clauss TM, Dove AD, Arnold JE. Hematologic disorders of fish. The Veterinary Clinics of North America. 2008;**11**(3):445-462

[5] Ali H, V. Rani V. Effect of phosalone on haematological indices in the tilapia, *Oreochromis mossambicus*. Turkish Journal of Veterinary and Animal Sciences. 2009;**33**(5):407-411. DOI: 10.3906/vet-0804-43

[6] Burgos-Aceves MA, Lionetti L, Faggio C. Multidisciplinary haematology as prognostic device in environmental and xenobiotic stress-induced response in fish. The Science of the Total Environment. 2019;**670**:1170-1183. DOI: 10.1016/j.scitotenv.2019.03.275

[7] Northrop-Clewes CA, Thurnham DI. Biomarkers for the differentiation of anemia and their clinical usefulness. Journal of Blood Medicine. 2013;**4**:11-22. DOI: 10.2147/JBM.S29212

[8] Luskova V. Annual cycles and normal values of hematological parameters in fishes. Acta scientiarum naturalium Academiae Scientiarum Bohemicae Brno. 1997;**31**(5):70-78

[9] Fazio F. Fish hematology analysis as an important tool of aquaculture: A review. Aquaculture. 2019;**500**:237-242. DOI: 10.1016/j.aquaculture.2018.10.030

[10] Tucker CS, Francis-Floyd R, Beleau MH. Nitrite-induced anemia in channel catfish, *Ictalurus punctatus* rafinesque. Bulletin of Environmental Contamination and Toxicology. 1989;**43**(2):295-301

[11] Da Costa OTF, Dos Santos FDJ, Mendonça FLP, Fernandes MN. Susceptibility of the Amazonian fish, *Colossoma macropomum* (Serrasalminae), to short-term exposure to nitrite. Aquaculture. 2004;**232**:627-636. DOI: 10.1016/S0044-8486(03)00524-6

[12] Zhelev Z, Mollova D, Boyadziev P. Morphological and hematological parameters of *Carassius Gibelio* (Pisces: Gyprinidae) in conditions of anthropogenic pollution in southern Bulgaria. Use of hematological parameters as biomarkers. Trakia Journal of Sciences. 2016;**1**:1-15. DOI: 10.15547/tjs.2016.01.001

[13] Fedeli D, Carloni M, Falcioni G. Oxidative damage in trout erythrocyte in response to "in vitro" copper exposure. Marine Environmental Research. 2010;**69**(3):172-177. DOI: 10.1016/j.marenvres.2009.10.001

[14] Georgieva E, Arnaudov A, Velcheva I. Clinical, hematological and morphological studies on ex situ induced copper intoxication in Crucian carp (*Carassius gibelio*). Journal of Central European Agriculture. 2010;**11**(2):165-171

[15] Som M, Kundu N, Bhattacharyya S, Homechaudhuri S. Evaluation of

hemopoietic responses in *Labeo rohita* Hamilton following acute copper toxicity. Toxicological and Environmental Chemistry. 2009;**91**(1):87-98. DOI: 10.1080/02772240801990700

[16] Garofano JS, Hirshfield HI. Peripheral effects of cadmium on the blood and head kidney in the brown bullhead (*Ictalurus nebulosus*). Bulletin of the Environmental Contamination Toxicology. 1982;**28**(5):552-556. DOI: 10.1007/BF01605583

[17] Kondera E, Witeska M. Cadmium and copper reduce hematopoietic potential in common carp (*Cyprinus carpio* L.) head kidney. Fish Physiology and Biochemistry. 2013;**39**(4):755-764. DOI: 10.1007/s10695-012-9738-6

[18] Arnaudov AD, Velcheva IG, Tomova ES. Influence of copper and zinc on the erythrocyte-metric parameters of *Carassius gibelio* (PISCES, CYPRINIDAE) I. influence of copper on the erythrocyte-metric parameters of *Carassius gibelio* (PISCES, CYPRINIDAE). Bulgarian Journal of Agricultural Science. 2008;**14**(6):557-563

[19] Akahori A, Jóźwiak Z, Gabryelak T, Gondko R. Effect of zinc on carp (*Cyprinus carpio* L.) erythrocytes. Comparative Biochemistry and Physiology Part C. 1999;**123**(3):209-215. DOI: 10.1016/s0742-8413(00)00161-4

[20] Gabryelak T, Filipiak A, Brichon G. Effects of zinc on lipids of erythrocytes from carp (*Cyprinus carpio* L.) acclimated to different temperatures. Comparative Biochemistry and Physiology Part C: Pharmacology, Toxicology and Endocrinology. 2000;**127**(3):335-343. DOI: 10.1016/s0742-8413(00)00161-4

[21] Witeska M, Kościuk B. The changes in common carp blood after short-term zinc exposure. Environmental Science and Pollution Research. 2003;**10**(5):284-286. DOI: 10.1065/espr2003.07.161

[22] Tomova E, Arnaudov A, Velcheva I. Effects of zinc on morphology of erythrocytes and spleen in *Carassius gibelio*. Journal of Environmental Biology. 2008;**29**(6):897-902

[23] Arnaudov A, Velcheva I, Tomova E. Changes in the erythrocytes indexes of *Carassius gibelio* (Pisces, Cyprinidae) under the influence of zinc. Biotechnology and Biotechnological Equipment. 2009;**23**(supl. 1):167-169. DOI: 10.1080/13102818.2009.10818391

[24] Tomova E, Velcheva I, Arnaudov A. Influence of copper and zinc on the erythrocyte-metric parameters of *Carassius gibelio* (PISCES, CYPRINIDAE) II. Influence of zinc on the erythrocyte-metric parameters of *Carassius gibelio* (PISCES, CYPRINIDAE). Bulgarian Journal of Agricultural Science. 2009;**15**(3):183-188

[25] Nakagawa H, Nakagawa K, Sato T. Evaluation of erythrocyte 5-aminolevulinic acid dehydratase activity in the blood of carp *Cyprinus carpio* as an indicator in fish with water lead pollution. Fisheries Science. 1995;**61**(1):91-95

[26] Caldwell C, Phillips KA. Hematological effects in rainbow trout subjected to a chronic sublethal concentration of lead. In: Kennedy C, Mackinlay D, editors. Fish Response to Toxic Environments: Symposium Proceedings International Congress on the Biology of F. Bethesda, MD: American Fisheries Society; 1998. pp. 61-62

[27] Arnaudova D, Boyadjieva-Doychinova D, Arnaudov A. Changes in blood cells of carp (*Cyprinus carpio*

L.) under the influence of increasing concentrations of lead. Scientific works of the Union of Scientists–Plovdiv Series B: Technics and Technologies. 2019;**17**:188-192

[28] Witeska M, Kondera E, Szymańska M, Ostrysz M. Hematological changes in common carp (*Cyprinus carpio* L.) after short-term Lead (Pb) exposure. Polish Journal of Environmental Studies. 2010;**19**(4):825-828

[29] Arnaudov A, Arnaudova D. Changes in blood cells of carp (*Cyprinus carpio* L.) under the influence of increasing concentrations of nickel. Scientific works of the Union of Scientists–Plovdiv Series B: Technics and Technologies. 2017;**14**:210-213

[30] De Luca G, Gugliotta T, Parisi G, Romano P, Geraci A, Romano O, et al. Effects of nickel on human and fish red blood cells. Bioscience Reports. 2007;**27**(4):265-273. DOI: 10.1007/s10540-007-9053-0

[31] Parthipan P, Muniyan M. Effect of heavy metal nickel on hematological parameters of fresh water fish, *Cirrhinus mrigala*. Journal of Environment and Current Life Science. 2013;**1**:46-55. DOI: 10.13140/2.1.3256.2883

[32] Moosavi MJ, Shamushaki VAJ. Effect of sub-acute exposure to nickel on hematological and biochemical indices in gold fish (*Carassius auratus*). Journal of Clinical Toxicology. 2015;**5**(1):228. DOI: 10.4172/2161-0495.1000228

[33] Elahee KB, Bhagwant S. Hematological and gill histopathological parameters of three tropical fish species from a polluted lagoon on the west coast of Mauritius. Ecotoxicology and Environmental Safety. 2007;**68**(3):361-371. DOI: 10.1016/j.ecoenv.2006.06.003

[34] Arnaudova D, Arnaudov A, Tomova E. Selected hematological indices of freshwater fish from Studen Kladenetsh reservoir. Bulgarian Journal of Agricultural Science. 2008;**14**(2):244-250

[35] Omar WA, Zaghloul KH, Abdel-Khalek AA, Abo-Hegab S. Genotoxic effects of metal pollution in two fish species, *Oreochromis niloticus* and *Mugil cephalus*, from highly degraded aquatic habitats. Mutation Research, Genetic Toxicology and Environmental Mutagenesis. 2012;**746**(1):7-14. DOI: 10.1016/j.mrgentox.2012.01.013

[36] Fedonenko O, Yesipova N, Sharamok T. The accumulation of heavy metals and cytometric characteristics features of red blood cells in different ages of carp fish from Zaporozhian reservoir. International Letters of Natural Sciences. 2016;**53**:72-79. DOI: 10.18052/www.scipress.com/ILNS.53.72

[37] Tahir R, Ghaffar A, Abbas G, Turabi TH, Kausar S, Xiaoxia D, et al. Pesticide induced hematological, biochemical and genotoxic changes in fish: A review. Agrobiological records. 2021;**3**:41-57. DOI: 10.17957/IJAB/17.3.14.1016

[38] Sinha BK, Gour JK, Singh MK, Nigam AK. Effects of pesticides on haematological parameters of fish: Recent updates. Journal of Scientific Research. *2022*;**66**(1):270-283. DOI: 10.37398/JSR.2022.660129

[39] Mikula P, Modra H, Nemethova D, Groch L, Svobodova Z. Effects of subchronic exposure to LASSO MTX®(alachlor 42% W/V) on hematological indices and histology of the common carp, *Cyprinus carpio* L. Bulletin of Environmental Contamination and Toxicology.

2008;**81**(5):475-479. DOI: 10.1007/s00128-008-9500-z

[40] Dogan D, Can C. Hematological, biochemical, and behavioral responses of *Oncorhynchus mykiss* to dimethoate. Fish Physiology and Biochemistry. 2011;**37**(4):951-958. DOI: 10.1007/s10695-011-9492-1

[41] Ghaffar A, Hussain R, Abbas G, Khan R, Akram K, Latif H, et al. Assessment of genotoxic and pathologic potentials of fipronil insecticide in *Labeo rohita* (Hamilton, 1822). Toxin Reviews. 2019. DOI: 10.1080/15569543.2019.1684321

[42] Hii YS, Lee MY, Chuah TS. Acute toxicity of organochlorine insecticide endosulfan and its effect on behaviour and some hematological parameters of Asian swamp eel (*Monopterus albus*, Zuiew). Pesticide Biochemistry and Physiology. 2007;**89**(1):46-53. DOI: 10.1016/j.pestbp.2007.02.009

[43] Ambreen F, Javed M. Pesticide mixture induced DNA damage in peripheral blood erythrocytes of freshwater Fish, *Oreochromis niloticus*. Pakistan Journal of Zoology. 2018;**50**(1):339-346

[44] Van Apeldoorn ME, Van Egmond HP, Speijers GJ, Bakker GJ. Toxins of cyanobacteria. Molecular Nutrition & Food Research. 2007;**51**(1):7-60. DOI: 10.1002/mnfr.200600185

[45] Zhang X, Xie P, Li D, Shi Z. Hematological and plasma biochemical responses of crucian carp (*Carassius auratus*) to intraperitoneal injection of extracted microcystins with the possible mechanisms of anemia. Toxicon. 2007;**v49(8)**:1150-1157. DOI: 10.1016/j.toxicon.2007.02.009

[46] Zhou W, Liang H, Zhang X. Erythrocyte damage of crucian carp (*Carassius auratus*) caused by microcystin-LR: In vitro study. Fish Physiology and Biochemistry. 2012;**38**(3):849-858. DOI: 10.1007/s10695-011-9572-2

[47] Navrátil S, Palíková M, Vajcová V. The effect of pure microcystin LR and biomass of blue-green algae on blood indices of carp (*Cyprinus carpio* L.). Acta Veterinaria Brno. 1998;**67**(4):273-279. DOI: 10.2754/avb199867040265

[48] Vosylienė MZ. The effect of heavy metals on haematological indices of fish (survey). Acta Zoologica Lituanica. 1999;**9**(2):76-82. DOI: 10.1080/13921657.1999.10512290

[49] Nikinmaa M. (2001). Haemoglobin function in vertebrates: Evolutionary changes in cellular regulation in hypoxia. Respiration Physiology. 2001;**128**(3):317-329. DOI: 10.1016/s0034-5687(01)00309-7

Chapter 9

Behaviour of a Sialo-Oligosaccharide from Glycophorin in Teleost Red Blood Cell Membranes

Takahiko Aoki

Abstract

Glycophorins (GPs) in red blood cell (RBC) membranes of carp (*Cyprinus carpio* L.) exhibit bacteriostatic activity against various gram-negative and gram-positive bacteria including fish pathogens. This physiological property also exists in the GPs of yellow tail (*Seriola quinqueradiata*) and red sea bream (*Pagrus major*). Thus, we concluded that this antimicrobial activity is not confined to these teleost species but can be found in all fish. This bacteriostatic activity is caused by the sialo-oligosaccharide from these teleost GPs. Only the *N*-glycolylneuraminic acid (NeuGc) form of sialic acid was detected in the carp. Using NMR and GC–MS, we determined that the structure of the bacteriostatic sialo-oligosaccharide from carp was NeuGcα2→6 (Fucα1→4) (Glcα1→3) Galβ1→4GalNAc-ol. The bacteriostatic activity of this mono sialyl oligosaccharide is due to the property of the lectin receptor. It is supposed that some lectin-like proteins exist on the surface of gram-positive bacteria or the flagellum of gram-negative bacteria. Based on the electron microscope observations, teleost GPs containing the sialo-oligosaccharide are released from RBC membranes and then adsorbed onto the surface or the flagellum of invading bacteria in the blood.

Keywords: teleost, carp, yellow tail, red sea bream, red blood cell membranes, glycophorin, antibiotic activity, oligosaccharide, sialic acid

1. Introduction

The blood of mammals such as humans, as well as birds, reptiles and teleosts, contains red blood cells (RBCs; erythrocytes). Human RBCs are the most commonly studied cells for structural and physiological analysis. While human RBCs are approximately 7 μm in diameter, and their centre has a dented discoid shape, teleost RBCs are slightly larger than human RBCs, have nuclei, and have a not dented orbicularity or oval shape (**Figure 1**) [1, 2].

Studies on biological membranes normally use human RBCs since they have no nuclei and are easy to obtain for RBC membrane preparation after the hemolysis procedure. For the preparation of RBC membrane proteins, it is necessary to use detergents for the solubilization of the phospholipid bilayer. Fairbanks et al. [3]

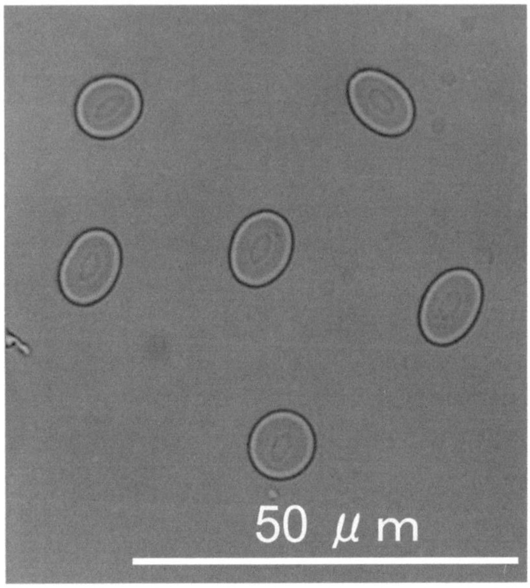

Figure 1.
Carp red blood cells (×500).

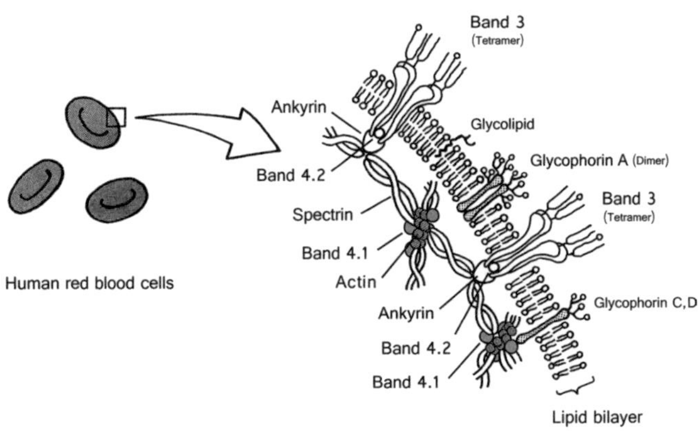

Figure 2.
Illustration showing the location of band 3 and GPs in human RBC membranes. This illustration is based on several reviews [4–6]. According to Lux [4], the location of substoichiometric proteins remains unclear. In this illustration, these glycoproteins are omitted, the actin junctional complex (4.1R complex) is simplified, and the topology of band 3 and glycophorins is defined.

developed a method in which RBC membranes were solubilized by sodium dodecyl sulfate (SDS), and then the extracted membrane proteins were separated on polyacrylamide gel by electrophoresis (SDS–PAGE). Using the method of SDS-PAGE, major membrane proteins and glycoproteins in RBCs could be detected on SDS gels. However, minor components in human RBC membranes such as substoichiometric proteins (e.g., CD44, CD47, Lu, Kell, Duffy), are not detected clearly on SDS-gels [4]. **Figure 2** shows a schematic drawing of the human RBC membrane structure, with reference to reviews of the RBC membrane skeleton [4–6].

2. Membrane proteins of the human and teleost RBC membranes

By using SDS–PAGE, membrane proteins could be detected on SDS gels by staining with Coomassie brilliant blue (CBB). **Figure 3** Lane 2 shows typical human RBC membrane proteins separated by SDS–PAGE using the method of Laemmli [7], which was later improved by Fairbanks et al. [3]. The number depicts the nomenclature of each cell membrane protein according to Fairbanks et al. [3]. Band 3, band 4.1 and band 4.2 are currently called the proper names. Band 3, which is an anion transporter as AE1, is detectable as a diffuse band on the SDS-gel due to the microheterogeneity of the oligosaccharides attached to GPs [8]. Although Band 3 is a glycoprotein, it is detectable on SDS gel using protein staining with CBB. This is attributed to a small amount of oligosaccharides in band 3 compared to the protein amount. Approximately 7% of carbohydrates have been contained in Band 3, and contributes to 10% of the total membrane carbohydrate [9].

We examined the membrane proteins in the RBCs of carp (*Cyprinus carpio* L.) (**Figure 3** Lane 5), yellow tail (*Seriola quinqueradiata*) and red sea bream (*Pagrus major*) (**Figure 4** Lanes 2 and 5) by SDS–PAGE. By comparison with molecular mass standards, the prominent protein bands of carp, yellow tail and red sea bream RBC membranes were band 3, band 1 (spectrin α chain) and band 2 (spectrin β chain), and band 4.1, band 5 (actin) and band 7 were designated for human membrane proteins. The general profiles of the CBB stain pattern on the SDS-gels were not strikingly different compared to that of human RBC membranes.

In the red sea bream, the presence of lipids led to broadening of the low-molecular-weight bands (**Figure 4** Lane 5). In the yellow tail membranes, spectrin bands were fainter than those in other fish species (**Figure 4** Lane 2). It is suggested that the cysteine protease, cathepsin L, hydrolysed these cytoskeletal fibers. Ahimbisibwe et al. [10] reported the presence of cathepsin L in the RBC membranes of several

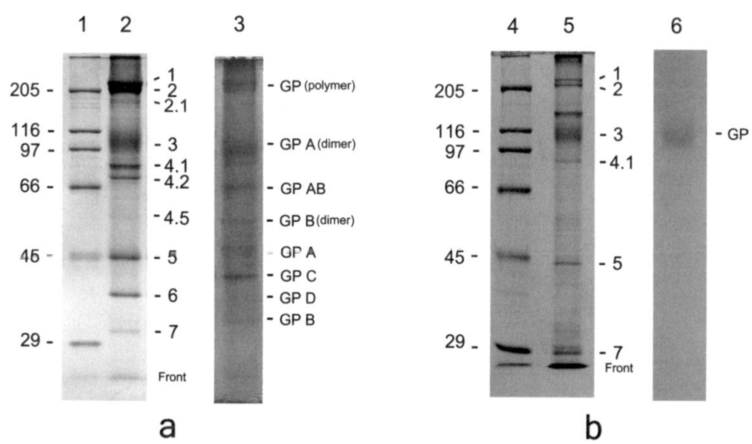

Figure 3.
SDS-PAGE of carp and human RBC membranes. (a) Coomassie brilliant blue R-250 (CBB)- and PAS-stained human RBC membranes. Lane 1, CBB-stained molecular mass standards: myosin (205 kDa); β-galactosidase (116 kDa); phosphorylase b (97 kDa); bovine albumin (66 kDa); egg albumin (45 kDa); and carbonic anhydrase (29 kDa). Lane 2, CBB-stained human RBC membranes. Lane 3, PAS-stained human RBC membranes. (b) CBB- and PAS-stained carp RBC membranes. Lane 4, CBB-stained molecular mass standards. Lane 5, CBB-stained carp RBC membranes. Lane 6, PAS-stained carp RBC membranes. GP, glycophorin. The number denotes the membrane protein designations for human RBC membrane proteins. Approximately 30 μg of membrane protein were applied per lane.

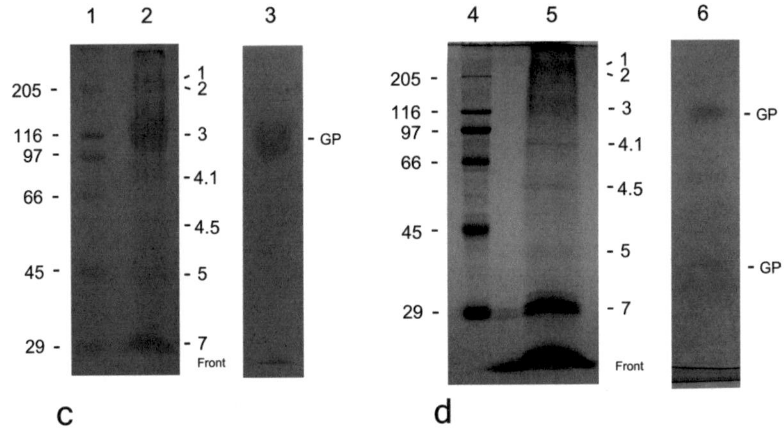

Figure 4.
SDS-PAGE of yellow tail and red sea bream RBC membranes. (a) CBB- and PAS-stained yellow tail RBC membranes. Lane 1, CBB-stained molecular mass standards. Lane 2, CBB-stained yellow tail RBC membranes. Lane 3, PAS-stained yellow tail RBC membranes. (b) CBB- and PAS-stained red sea bream RBC membranes. Lane 4, CBB-stained molecular mass standards. Lane 5, CBB-stained red sea bream RBC membranes. Lane 6, PAS-stained red sea bream RBC membranes. GP, glycophorin. The number denotes the membrane protein designations for human RBC membrane proteins. Approximately 30 μg of membrane protein were applied per lane.

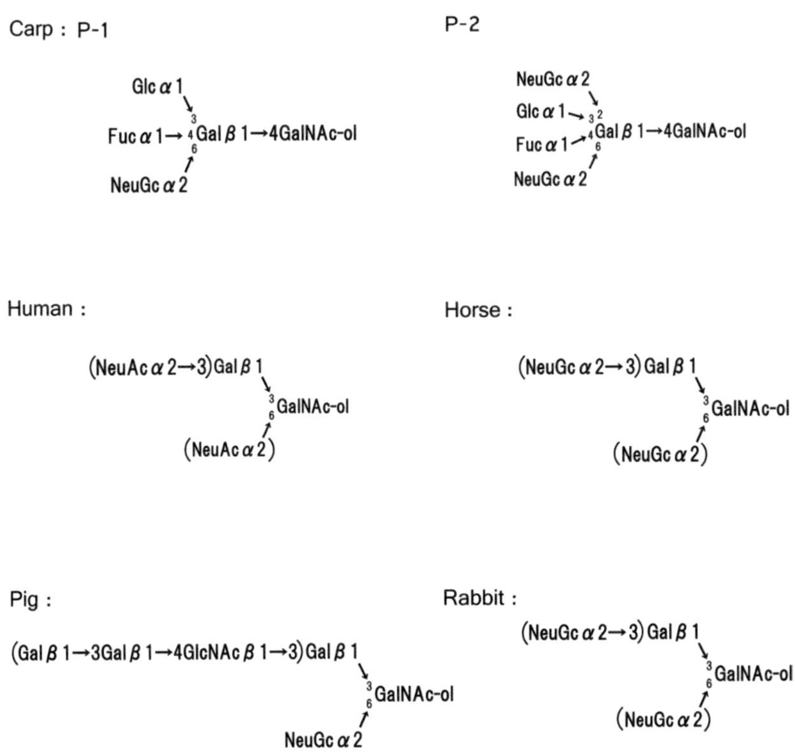

Figure 5.
Basic structures of O-linked oligosaccharides of GPs of mammalian and carp origins.

teleosts (carp, amberjack and red sea bream), and the specific activity of cathepsin L was highest in the RBC membranes of amberjack, followed by carp and red sea bream. Aoki and Ueno [11] also reported that cathepsin L in mackerel muscle significantly hydrolysed myofibrils.

3. Glycophorins of human RBC membranes

Apart from the membrane proteins that Fairbanks et al. designated, glycophorins (GPs) exist as transmembrane glycoproteins that contain sialic acid. These sialo-oligosaccharide-rich glycoproteins are detectable on SDS-gels by staining with periodic acid-Schiff (PAS) reagent [3, 12]. **Figure 3** Lane 3 shows the nomenclature of human RBC membrane sialo-glycoproteins. These GPs are found in the RBC membranes of humans [13–16] and other mammals [17–20] and birds [21, 22]. In human RBC membranes, GP A (dimer) is observed below band 3 on SDS-gels (**Figure 3** Lane 3). GP A is a major component of red cell membrane glycoproteins. The electrophoretic migration of GP on SDS gels is relatively low when compared to other membrane proteins because GP is heavily glycosylated. Although the molecular mass of the other membrane proteins can be estimated by migration on SDS–PAGE, each GPs molecular mass cannot be estimated in this manner.

GPs C and D are thought to link to the band 4.1 protein and connect the cytoskeleton structure under the phospholipid bilayer [23–26]. These GPs C, D, and band 3 are associated with the cytoskeleton closely and contributed to the maintenance of the shape and mechanical properties of the RBC after passing through capillary vessels [27]. This information suggested that GPs C and D are anchored to the RBC membrane by the cytoskeleton. In contrast, it is believed that GPs A and B are not associated with the cytoskeleton, thus enabling them to be easily released from the RBC membrane [28].

While GP C and its shorter form, GP D, are antigenically distinct from GPs A and B. GP C carries several blood group antigens (Gerbich, Yus, Wb, Ana, Dha, and others) [29–31]. According to Podbielska et al. [32], O-linked oligosaccharides isolated from GP A carry the A, B, or H blood group antigen. Although these oligosaccharides reacted with ABH blood group antigens, the reaction was estimated at a relatively low level. Moreover, GP A-deficient RBCs did not clearly demonstrate the physiological role of GP A [33].

4. Glycoproteins of teleost RBC membranes

We examined the GPs in the RBCs of carp (**Figure 3** Lane 6), yellow tail and red sea bream (**Figure 4** Lanes 3 and 6) by SDS–PAGE under the same conditions as the human preparation, followed by staining with PAS reagent.

The PAS-stained bands in all teleost preparations were stained poorly in the same way as avian GPs [34]. The carp and yellow tail RBC membrane preparations yielded one major band on the SDS-gels (**Figures 3** Lane 6 and **4** Lane 3). The PAS stain pattern on the SDS-gels suggests that the carp and yellow tail RBC membranes had fewer forms of GP than the human RBC membrane. The main carp GP was located near the position of the carp and human band-3 proteins. In addition, the main carp GP was positioned near human GP A (dimer).

In the red sea bream, one major band and a faint band with lower molecular weight were observed (**Figure 4** Lane 6). Aoki et al. [35] detected some GP bands in rainbow trout preparation. There was one major band and two faint bands with lower molecular weights were detected. It was presumed that the major band was the GP dimer, while the faint band beneath the major band and the faint band with lower molecular weight were the incomplete polymer and monomer forms respectively. It is suggested that the major band in the red sea bream was a polymer form.

While membrane protein patterns (CBC-stained band patterns) are generally similar to those in humans, GP patterns (PAS-stained band patterns) are different in humans. These differences are caused by the components containing sialo-oligosaccharides.

5. Structure of a sialo-oligosaccharide from carp RBC membranes

We examined the amino acid composition of carp GP followed by the kind of sialic acid. While the amino acid composition was not strikingly different compared to that of human GP A, with the exception of valine, lysine and arginine, only the *N*-glycolylneuraminic acid (NeuGc) form of sialic acid was detected in the carp GP by TLC and a colorimetric method [36].

There are several reports on the sialic acid component of mammals sources of GP. In humans, GP contains *N*-acetylneuraminic acid (NeuAc), whereas the presence of NeuGc has been reported in GPs of horses [37], bovine [38], pig [39], and monkeys (*Macaca fuscata*) [19] and others. However, to date, little is known about sialic acid in teleost GPs. Compared to the sialic acids from nonhuman sources, this result suggested that teleosts contained the NeuGc, not as NeuAc. Interestingly, NeuGc has also been reported in the eggs of rainbow trout, chum salmon and land-locked cherry salmon [40].

The carbohydrate fraction of carp GP was separated into two components (P-1 and P-2) using a Glyco-Pak DEAE column with a continuous linear gradient of 0–100 mM NaCl. This fraction contained at least two kinds of O-linked oligosaccharides. Based on the chromatogram obtained using a NeuAc oligomer (α,2→8), the electro-negativity suggested that P-1 contained one sialic acid residue, whereas P-2 contained two residues [36].

We obtained *ca.* 190 μg P-1 and *ca.* 7.0 μg P-2 (as total carbohydrate) by HPLC from carp GP (*ca.* 4.0 mg protein). Using the graphite carbon column with ammonium bicarbonate in acetonitrile solution as an eluent, the yield of desalted oligosaccharide was satisfactory (P-1: *ca.* 90% and P-2: *ca.* 100%) [36].

These O-linked oligosaccharides (P-1 and P-2) were composed of glucose, galactose, fucose, *N*-acetylgalactosamine (GalNAc) and NeuGc. Using NMR and GC–MS, we determined that the structures of P-1 and P-2 were NeuGcα2→6(Fucα1→4)(Glcα1→3) Galβ1→4GalNAc-ol [41] and NeuGcα2→6(Fucα1→4)(Glcα1→3)(NeuGcα2→2) Galβ1→4GalNAc-ol, respectively (**Figure 5**). These O-linked oligosaccharides were unique to vertebrates with respect to the hexosamine and hexose linkages and their nonchain structure.

Human GPs contain O-linked sialo-oligosaccharides, and the structure of these oligosaccharides has been analysed [42]. The most commonly elucidated GP oligosaccharides from mammals sources are reported as below: tetra-saccharide core, NeuAcα2→3Galβ1→3(NeuAcα2→6)GalNAc-ol; tri-saccharide cores, Galβ1→3(NeuAcα2→6)GalNAc-ol or NeuAcα2→3Galβ1→3GalNAc-ol (**Figure 5**).

O-linked oligosaccharides containing NeuGc have also been reported among horse, pig, and rabbit GPs, and the most commonly reported structure is a trisaccharide, Galβ1→3(NeuGcα2→6) GalNAc-ol [20]. Other derivatives are synthesized by attaching NeuGc and Gal residues to the trisaccharide core [28].

Although Glc residue in O-linked oligosaccharides has not been reported to detect in mammalian [20] and chicken GPs [43], Guérardel et al. [44] reported that *O*-glycans synthesized by nematodes contained the Glc residue, whereas the Fuc residue was detected in the O-linked oligosaccharides of human GP A [32].

From the NMR spectra obtained using the asialo P-1 fraction, the characterized proton signals revealed an overall downfield shift in the resonance of αGlc and αFuc, except for the H-1 signals [41]. This O-linked oligosaccharide indicates a globule form rather than chain-like structure. Furthermore, the linkage between Gal and GalNAc-ol is 1→4, unlike the 1→3 standard linkage for O-linked oligosaccharides. The 1→4 linkage of GalNAc is unique compared with other O-linked oligosaccharides of mammals sources of GP. Interestingly, the glycosidic linkage of xylan from the seaweed cell wall is the β1→3 unlike the standard β1→4 linkage of xylan from land plants [45]. It seems possible to detect the β1→4 linkage of GalNAc in marine organisms.

6. Physiological activity of GPs from carp, yellow tail and red sea bream

We performed a sensitivity test using GP preparations from the carp RBC membranes. The sensitivity test for the growth of test bacteria was performed using the disc-plate method [36, 46]. All of the test bacteria (gram-positive bacteria: *Micrococcus luteus* and *Bacillus subtilis*, gram-negative bacteria: *Aeromonas hydrophila*, *Vibrio anguillarum*, *Pseudomonas fluorescens*, *Edwardsiella tarda* and *Escherichia coli*) formed inhibition zones around the paper disc containing the GP fraction (**Figure 6**). For *E. tarda*, the inhibition zones were observed over a light box to discern the production of FeS from SS agar medium (**Figure 6**f). *M. luteus and E. coli* produced yellow pigments and white pigments, respectively (**Figure 6**d and g). While the outer zone of *M. luteus and E. coli* did not produce pigments, the inner zone represented growth inhibition. In contrast, the inhibition zone was not formed around the paper discs containing PBS (**Figure 6**g).

To clarify the physiological activity of teleost fish GPs other than those from carp, we performed a sensitivity test for the growth of *M. luteus* using GP preparations from the RBC membranes of yellow tail and red sea bream (**Figure 7**) [47]. These results showed that not only carp GP preparations but also yellow tail and red sea bream GPs had antibiotic activities.

Compared with the profile of forming an inhibition zone, these results also suggested that the yellow tail or red sea bream GPs have a broad-spectrum antibiotic activity similar to that of carp GP. While carp are freshwater fish, yellow tail and red sea bream are marine red-flesh fish and white-flesh fish, respectively. Thus, it is assumed that the antimicrobial activity of sialo-origosaccharide from GP is not confined to these teleost species but can be found in all fish.

Then, we examined which GP fraction demonstrates bacteriostatic activity by using a sensitivity test [36]. The carp RBC membrane preparation, GP preparation, carbohydrate and P-1 fractions also exhibited bacteriostatic activity (**Figure 8**a–f). The P-2 fraction exhibited bacteriostatic activity within the area of the disc paper (**Figure 8**e and f). In contrast, the inhibition zones were not observed using the GP

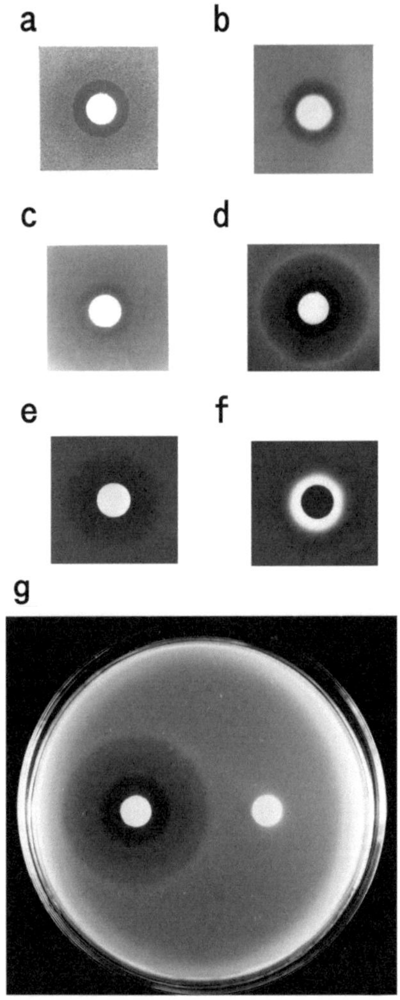

Figure 6.
Sensitivity test of the carp GP fraction for the growth of several bacteria by the disc-plate method. (a) Carp GP fraction (ca. 15 μg·protein/disc) to B. subtilis; (b) GP fraction (ca. 15 μg·protein/disc) to A. hydrophila; (c) GP fraction (ca. 15 μg·protein/disc) to V. anguillarum; (d) GP fraction (ca. 15 μg·protein/disc) to M. luteus; (e) GP fraction (ca. 15 μg·protein/disc) to P. fluorescens; (e) GP fraction (ca. 15 μg·protein/disc) to P. fluorescens; (f) GP fraction (ca. 15 μg·protein/disc) to E. tarda; (g) GP fraction (ca. 15 μg·protein/disc) to E. coli (left disc; GP fraction, right disc; PBS). A paper disc (8 mm diameter) containing each fraction was placed on the medium and incubated at 20°C. After 24–48 h, the inhibition zone was observed on each plate.

fraction that lacked sialic acid or the human GP. These results suggest that the test bacteria are sensitive to monosialyl-oligosaccharides from teleost GPs.

Based on electron microscope observations [36], the carp GP molecules attach to the flagellum of *V. anguillarum* rather than the cell itself (**Figure 9**a). Conversely, the GP molecules attach to the cell surface (contained cleavage line) on *M. luteus* (**Figure 9**b). Carp GP exists with the size of various molecules and has a diameter of 40–220 nm from TEM images (**Figure 9**c-3). It seems that the smallest GP molecules selectively possessed bacteriostatic activity.

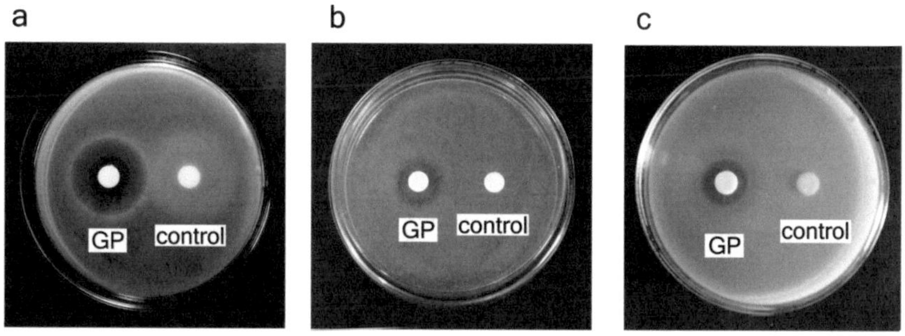

Figure 7.
Sensitivity test for M. luteus by the disc-plate method. (a) GP preparation from carp (ca. 15 μg protein/disc). GP, carp GP; control, PBS; (b) GP preparation from yellow tail (ca. 10 μg protein/disc). GP, yellow tail GP; control, PBS; (c) GP preparation from red sea bream (ca. 10 μg protein/disc). GP, red sea bream GP; control, PBS.

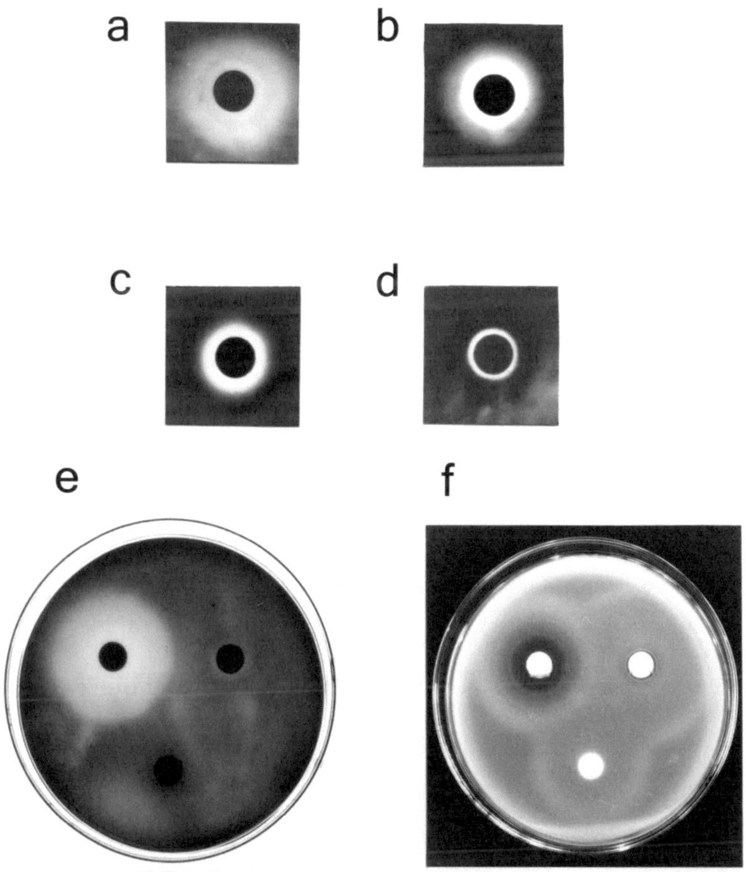

Figure 8.
Sensitivity test for the growth of E. tarda and M. luteus. (a) Carp RBC membranes (ca. 5 mg·protein/disc); (b) carp GP fraction without streptomycin treatment (ca. 17 μg·protein/disc); (c) carp GP fraction (ca. 15 μg·protein/disc); (d) carbohydrate fraction from carp GP (ca. 4 μg/disc); (e, f) P-1 and P-2 fractions (ca. 8 μg/disc each); upper left disc, P-1; upper right disc, P-2; lower disc, PBS. (a–e) Plates containing E. tarda; (f) plate containing M. luteus.

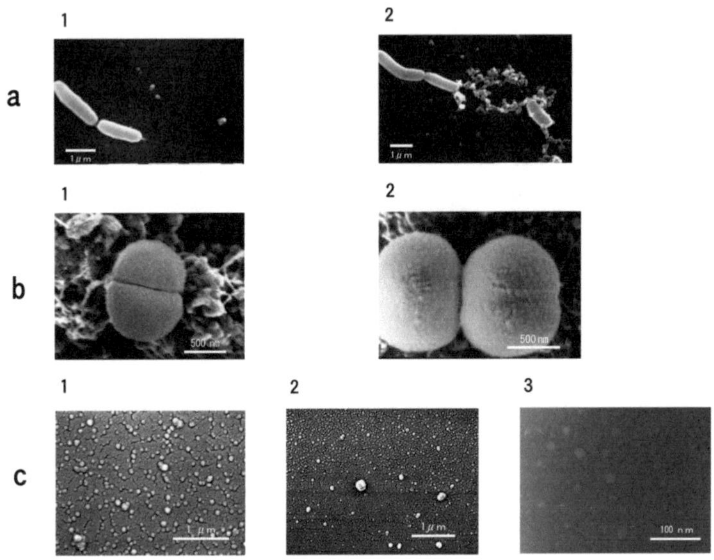

Figure 9.
Electron microscope images of the bacteria and carp GP. (a) V. anguillarum and carp GP. 1, V. anguillarum without carp GP; 2, V. anguillarum with carp GP. An equal volume of glycophorin solution (ca. 0.4 μg·protein/20 μL) was added to the cell suspension (ca. 3 × 10^6 cfu/20 μL) at 25°C. (b) M. luteus and carp GP. 1, M. luteus without carp GP; 2, M. luteus with carp GP. An equal volume of glycophorin solution (ca. 0.4 μg·protein/20 μL) was added to the cell suspension (ca. 3 × 10^6 cfu/20 μL) at 25°C. (c) Carp GP. 1, SEM image under the same conditions of V. anguillarum with carp GP; 2, SEM image under the same conditions of M. luteus with carp GP; 3, TEM image.

7. Behaviour of a sialo-oligosaccharide from GP in RBC membranes

These bacteriostatic activities of teleost GP are caused by the contained monosialyl-oligosaccharide and are attributed to the property of the lectin receptor. It is supposed that some lectin-like proteins exist on the surface of gram-positive bacteria or the component of flagellum of gram-negative bacteria. Based on the obtained observations, (1) the teleost GPs are released from RBC membranes and aggregated with each other by hydrophobic areas within the protein moiety of GP. (2) The sialo-oligosaccharides are exposed on the outer layer of the aggregated GP molecules. (3) Aggregated GP molecules are adsorbed onto the surface or the flagellum of invading bacteria in the blood plasma. (4) The bacteria attached to GP molecules will be led to a bacteriostatic state (**Figure 10**) [28].

The bacteriostatic activity of sialo-oligosaccharides from carp GP is attributed to pentose formation. This may be related to the bacteriostatic activity caused by the penta- or hexa-saccharides obtained from chitin [48]. In the bacteriostatic reaction by teleost GP, it is supposed that the size of the oligosaccharide corresponds to that of the cleft occurs in the lectin-like protein and also might contribute to the negative charge of sialic acid. In teleost blood, IgG does not exist unlike human blood, and other antibodies exist at low levels [49]. It is suggested that GP may exist as a substitute for antibodies such as IgG in teleost blood on the immune system. Although the physiological function of human GP has not yet been clarified, the structure of human GP's O-linked tetra-oligosaccharide is a simpler form than that of carp's pentose. And NeuAc in human GP is also simpler than carp's NeuGc. IgG is considered a major component in the human immune system, and the bacteriostatic activity of human GPs has been lost in the process of evolution.

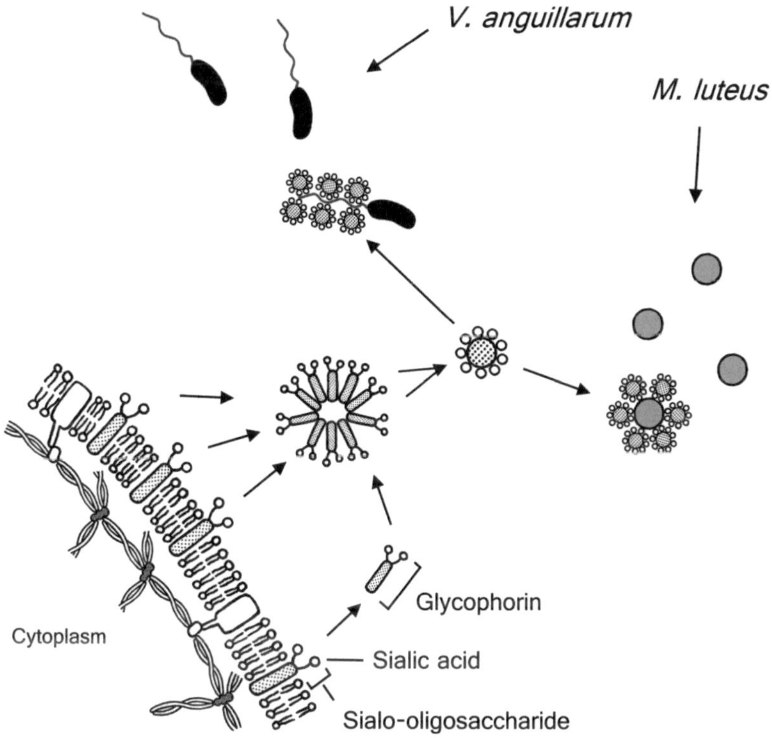

Figure 10.
Schematic representation of the teleost GP interaction with invading bacteria in fish blood.

Author details

Takavhiko Aoki
Laboratory of Quality in Marine Products, Graduate School of Bioresources, Mie University, Tsu, Mie, Japan

*Address all correspondence to: molnarba@inf.elte.hu

References

[1] Kakuno A, Sezaki K, Ikeda Y. Comparative hematology among 33 fish species of ostaryophysi. Bulletin of the National Research Institute of Fisheries Science. 1996;**8**:15-27

[2] Saitō K. Biochemical studies on the fish blood-XIV. On the mean corpuscular constant and shape of red corpuscule. Memoirs of Faculty of Fisheries Kagoshima University. 1959;7:192-197

[3] Fairbanks G, Steck TL, Wallach DFH. Electrophoretic analysis of the major polypeptides of the human erythrocyte membrane. Biochemistry. 1971;**10**:2606-2617

[4] Lux SE IV. Anatomy of the red cell membrane skeleton: unanswered questions. Blood. 2016;**127**:187-199

[5] Burton NM, Bruce LJ. Modelling the structure of the red cell membrane. Biochemistry and Cell Biology. 2011;**89**:200-215

[6] Mohandas N, Gallagher PG. Red cell membrane: past, present, and future. Blood. 2008;**112**:3939-3948

[7] Laemmli UK. Cleavage of structural proteins during the assembly of the head of bacteriophage T4. Nature. 1970;**227**:680-685

[8] Tanner MJA. Molecular and cellular biology of the erythrocyte anion exchanger (AE 1). Seminars in Hematology. 1993;**30**:34-57

[9] Steck T. The organization of proteins in the human red blood cell membrane: a review. Journal of Cell Biology. 1974;**62**:1-19

[10] Ahimbisibwe JB, Inoue K, Aoki T. Detection of cathepsin L in red cell membranes from fish blood. Fisheries Science. 2010;**76**:155-159

[11] Aoki T, Ueno R. Involvement of cathepsins B and L in the post-mortem autolysis of mackerel muscle. Food Research International. 1997;**30**:585-591

[12] Doerner KC, White BA. Detection of glycoproteins separated by nondenaturing polyacrylamide gel electrophoresis using the periodic acid-Schiff stain. Analytical Biochemistry. 1990;**187**:147-150

[13] Cartron J-P, Colin Y, Kudo S, Fukuda M. Molecular genetics of human erythrocyte sialoglycoproteins glycophorins A, B, C, and D. In: Harris JR, editor. Blood Cell Biochemistry. Vol. 1. New York City: Springer USA; 1990. pp. 299-335

[14] Blanchard D. Human red cell glycophorins: biochemical and antigenic properties. Transfusion Medicine Reviews. 1990;**4**:170-186

[15] Chasis JA, Mohandas N. Red blood cell glycophorins. Blood. 1992;**80**:1869-1879

[16] Tanner MJA. Molecular and cellular biology of the erythrocyte anion exchanger (AE1). Seminars in Hematology. 1993;**30**:34-57

[17] Yamashita T, Murayama J, Utsumi H, Hamada A. Structural studies of O-glycosidic oligosaccharide units of dog erythrocyte glycophorin. Biochimica et Biophysica Acta. 1985;**839**:26-31

[18] Angel A-S, Grönberg G, Krotkiewski H, Lisowska E, Nilsson B. Structural analysis of the N-linked oligosaccharides from murine

glycophorin. Archives of Biochemistry and Biophysics. 1991;**291**:76-88

[19] Murayama J-I, Utsumi H, Hamada A. Amino acid sequence of monkey erythrocyte glycophorin MK. Its amino acid sequence has a striking homology with that of human glycophorin A. Biochimica et Biophysica Acta. 1989;**999**:273-280

[20] Krotkiewski H. The structure of glycophorins of animal erythrocytes. Glycoconjugate Journal. 1988;**5**:35-48

[21] Watts C, Wheeler KP. Partial separation of a sodium-dependent transport system for amino acids in avian erythrocyte membranes. FEBS Letters. 1978;**94**:241-244

[22] Dockham PA, Vidaver GA. Comparison of human and pigeon erythrocyte membrane proteins by one- and two-dimensional gel electrophoresis. Comparative Biochemistry and Physiology Part B. 1987;**87**:171-177

[23] Hemming NJ, Anstee DJ, Mawby WJ, Reid ME, Tanner MJA. Localization of the protein 4.1-binding site on human erythrocyte glycophorins C and D. Biochemical Journal. 1994;**299**:191-196

[24] Hemming NJ, Anstee DJ, Staricoff MA, Tanner MJA, Mohandas N. Identification of the membrane attachment sites for protein 4.1 in the human erythrocyte. Journal of Biological Chemistry. 1995;**270**:5360-5366

[25] Reid ME, Takakuwa Y, Conboy J, Tchernia G, Mohandas N. Glycophorin C content of human erythrocyte membrane is regulated by protein 4.1. Blood. 1990;**11**:2229-2234

[26] Alloisio N, Dalla Venezia N, Rana A, Andrabi K, Texier P, Gilsanz F, et al. Evidence that red blood cell protein p55 may participate in the skeleton-membrane linkage that involves protein 4.1 and glycophorin C. Blood. 1993;**82**:1323-1327

[27] Staricoff MA, Tanner MJA. Role of band 3 and glycophorin C in the maintenance of the shape and mechanical properties of the human red blood cell. Cellular & Molecular Biology Letters. 1996;**1**:151-161

[28] Aoki T. A comprehensive review of our current understanding of red blood cell (RBC) glycoproteins. Membranes. 2017;**7**:56-74

[29] Anstee DJ, Ridgwell K, Tanner MJA, Daniels GL, Parsons SF. Individuals lacking the Gerbich blood-group antigen have alterations in the human erythrocyte membrane sialoglycoproteins β and γ. Biochemical Journal. 1984;**221**:97-104

[30] Dahr W, Moulds J, Baumeister G, Moulds M, Kiedrowski S, Hummel M. Altered membrane sialoglycoproteins in human erythrocytes lacking the Gerbich blood group antigens. Biological Chemistry Hoppe-Seyler. 1985;**366**:201-211

[31] Lisowska E. Antigenic properties of human glycophorins – an update. In: Wu AM, editor. The Molecular Immunology of Complex Carbohydrates–2. Boston, MA: Springer USA; 2001. pp. 155-169

[32] Podbielska M, Fredriksson S-Å, Nilsson B, Lisowska E, Krotkiewski H. ABH blood group antigens in O-glycans of human glycophorin A. Archives of Biochemistry and Biophysics. 2004;**429**:145-153

[33] Lesley JB, Groves JD, Okubo Y, Thilaganathan B, Tanner JA. Altered

band 3 structure and function in glycophorin A- and B-deficient (M^kM^k) red blood cells. Blood. 1994;**84**:916-922

[34] Jackson RC. The exterior surface of the chicken erythrocyte. Journal of Biological Chemistry. 1975;**250**:617-622

[35] Aoki T, Fukai M, Ueno R. Glycoproteins in red cell membranes from carp and rainbow trout. Fisheries Science. 1996;**62**:498-499

[36] Aoki T, Chimura K, Nakao N, Mizuno Y. Isolation and characterization of glycophorin from carp red blood cell membranes. Membranes. 2014;**4**:491-508

[37] Fukuda K, Tomita M, Hamada A. Isolation and characterization of alkali-labile oligosaccharide units from horse glycophorin. Journal of Biochemistry. 1980;**87**:687-693

[38] Fukuda K, Kawashima I, Tomita M, Hamada A. Structural studies of the acidic oligosaccharide units from bovine glycophorin. Biochimica et Biophysica Acta. 1982;**717**:278-288

[39] Kawashima I, Fukuda K, Tomita M, Hamada A. Isolation and characterization of alkali-labile oligosaccharide units from porcine erythrocyte glycophorin. Journal of Biochemistry. 1982;**91**:865-872

[40] Sato C, Kitajima K, Tazawa I, Inoue Y, Inoue S, Troy FA II. Structural diversity in the α2→8-linked polysialic acid chains in salmonid fish egg glycoproteins. Journal of Biological Chemistry. 1993;**268**:23675-23684

[41] Aoki T, Chimura K, Sugiura H, Mizuno Y. Structure of a sialo-oligosaccharide from glycophorin in carp red blood cell membranes. Membranes. 2014;**4**:764-777

[42] Fukuda M, Lauffenburger M, Sasaki H, Rogers ME, Dell A. Structures of novel sialylated *O*-linked oligosaccharides isolated from human erythrocyte glycophorins. Journal of Biological Chemistry. 1987;**262**:11952-11957

[43] Duk M, Krotkiewski H, Stasyk TV, Lutsik-Kordovsky M, Syper D, Lisowska E. Isolation and characterization of glycophorin from nucleated (Chicken) erythrocytes. Archives of Biochemistry and Biophysics. 2000;**375**:111-118

[44] Guérardel Y, Balanzino L, Maes E, Leroy Y, Coddeville B, Oriol R, et al. The nematode *Caenorhabditis elegans* synthesizes unusial O-linked glycans: identification of glucose-substituted mucin-type O-glycans and short chondroitin-like oligosaccharides. Biochemical Journal. 2001;**357**:167-182

[45] Araki T, Aoki T, Kitamikado M. Isolation and Identification of a β-1,3-xylanase-producing bacterium. Nippon Suisan Gakkaishi. 1987;**53**:2077-2081

[46] Aoki T, Inoue T. Glycophorin in red blood cell membranes of healthy and diseased carp, *Cyprinus carpio* L. Journal of Fish Diseases. 2011;**34**:573-576

[47] Aoki T. Determination of the bacteriostatic activity of glycophorin preparations from red blood cell (RBC) membranes of yellow tail and red sea bream. Medical Research Archives. 2021;**9**. DOI: 10.18103/mra.v9i12.2613

[48] Uchida Y. Bacteriostatic activity and its application. (In Japanese). In: Chitin and Chitosan research association, editor. Application of Chitin, Chitosan. Tokyo, Japan; Gihodo Shuppan Co.; 1990. pp. 71-98.

[49] Wilson M, Bengtén E, Miller NW, Clem LW, Du Pasquier L, Warr GW. A novel chimeric Ig heavy chain from a teleost fish shares similarities to IgD. Proceedings of the National Academy of Sciences of the United States of America. 1997;**94**:4593-4597

Chapter 10

The Biological and Structural Organization of the Squid Brain

Diego Torrecillas Paula Lico

Abstract

Marine invertebrate models (squid, sepia, and octopus) made important contributions to description mammals' nervous system. Being a very simple nervous system relatively easy to be manipulated experimentally and visualized by simple microscope or magnifying glass, the giant synapses at stellate ganglion and the large synaptosomes prepared from the squid photoreceptor neurons served as an attractive model to Histology and Anatomy studies. This sophisticated nervous system has elucidated synaptic transmission in detail with their numerous proteins at presynaptic terminal, synaptic vesicle biogenesis, neurotransmitter secretion, vesicle recycling and, allowed the study of postsynaptic complex with their membranes receptors. However, there are few studies with biochemical and molecular approaches, which lead to a better understanding of their physiological functions and verify operation of such nervous system.

Keywords: nervous system, axons and giant synapses, synaptosomes and hnRNP proteins

1. Introduction

The brain is the control center that transmits the information of neurons to other groups of neurons. A single neuron can be affected simultaneously by excitatory and inhibitory stimuli from one axon or many other axons. Billions of neurons have different functions and constantly check the internal environment and external universe: light, touch, pressure, sound, balance, images, pain, emotion, consciousness. The nervous system from different external stimuli produces a continuous flow of information, memory, learning, and this conscious state throughout life seems infinite.

The nervous system of vertebrate is complex to be studied in individual or small groups of neurons. The cephalopods Coleoidea group (squid, sepia, and octopus), in addition to sea snails and nematodes, which contain few neurons and large structures, are relatively easy to manipulate experimentally and contributed to most of the current knowledge about the nervous system.

In general, these studies can be applicable to nervous system complexes, such as the human system. For example, mammals have a complexity of the Neuropil, an area composed of mostly unmyelinated axons, dendrites, and glial cell processes.

For few (μ^2) at Neuropil mammals, we find hundreds of bud's terminals with their corresponding dendritic spines and pre-postsynaptic terminals, where pointing them out individually would be a difficult task.

It was noticed that the Neuropil from squid nervous system also has many pre-postsynaptic terminals such as a mammal. However, these are much larger in the squid nervous system and allow different types of experimental manipulations. In fact, light microscopy cannot resolve synaptic densities and synaptic vesicles, but the active zones in synapses can be observed easily from squid nervous system using low-power electron microscopy.

Thus, the squid nervous system with giant synapses and giant axon system have contributed to the current knowledge of Electrophysiology, Molecular Biology, and Biochemistry and allowed to verify the synaptic transmission and synaptic plasticity.

2. Nature history of *Doryteuthis SSP*: in the South and North Atlantic

According to the classification by Young [1], cephalopod can be grouped in the subclasses Nautiloidea (nautiluses) and Coleoidea (all the others) or in the general morphology to include in taxonomic descriptions [2].

During the summer in the South and North Atlantic, the mature specimens of *Doryteuthis plei* or *Doryteuthis pealeii* (or *Doryteuthis ssp*) were collected with supports of Marine Biology Center at University of São Paulo (CEBIMar-USP) and Marine Biological Laboratory (MBL) at Woods Hole, US, respectively.

The squid survives chasing food by capturing prey and escaping predators. An ability to accelerate quickly and make sudden changes in the direction of swimming help them to avoid danger. This agility is ensured by the sophisticated nervous system [3, 4] specialized for propellant jets: that pull the water into mantle and then, with the aid of a muscular body wall, which is rapidly contracted, the water is expelled, thus propelling it through the water.

To obtain this muscle contraction result, the squid requires a nervous system that can conduct signals with great speed throughout the body. The optic lobe or "brain" located on each side of the squid head is the control center that transmits the information to the chain of giant nerve cells in the mantle (**Figure 1a**).

The giant axon can reach 10 cm in length and is about one hundred times than the axon diameter of mammal [5, 6]. The giant axon model made important contributions to the description of axoplasmatic flow mechanisms [7], ion transport across the plasma membrane [8], and neurotransmission [9], and also allowed micro-injections using specific antibodies such a tool for the study of molecules involved in the synaptic function [10, 11]. In addition, the neuronal system contributed to discovery that mRNAs are present in the presynaptic region [12, 13] and new proteins synthesis occurs locally in this region [14].

Here, the stellate ganglion and the large synaptosome from photoreceptor neurons were isolated from squid nervous system and showed a biological and structural organization of brain by biochemical and immunohistochemistry studies.

3. Ultrastructure: giant synapse

Intact stellate ganglion in the mantle was removed (**Figure 1b** see in pin). The stellate ganglion in seawater can be observed by glass magnification (**Figure 1c**). In more

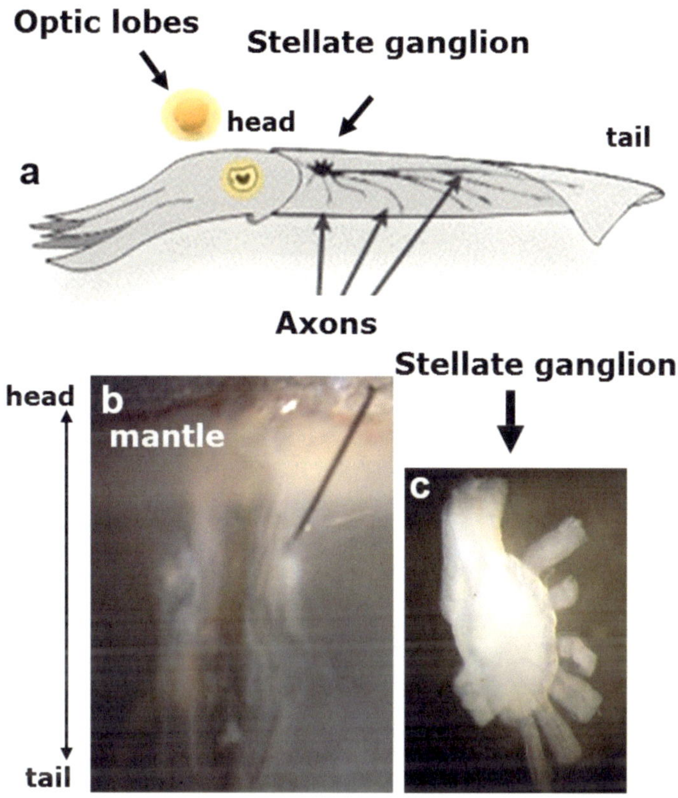

Figure 1.
The optic lobes and stellate ganglion with giant nerve fibers. a) Illustration shows a squid animal model with optic lobes on each side of head and stellate ganglion with chain of giant nerve cells on each side of the midline in the mantle. b) The stellate ganglion in mantle (seen in pin). c) The stellate ganglion visualized in seawater with glass vision 10x magnification.

detail, the presynaptic axon (Pre), postsynaptic axon (Post) and giant nerve fibers (Ax) are seen in **Figure 2a**.

In light microscopy, cross-sectional region from stellate ganglion shows synaptic contact region between the pre- and postsynaptic terminal at giant synapse when visualized by H&E staining (**Figure 2b**).

Low-power electron micrograph of same region from stellate ganglion shows synaptic densities and clustering of synaptic vesicles that can be observed in the active zones (**Figure 3**). The presynaptic (Pre) terminal is lighter than the postsynaptic (Post) terminal and can be characterized by the presence of synaptic vesicles. In the contact areas, the postsynaptic sends digitiform processes and forms the active zones in the limits of interaction between presynaptic terminals. The electron micrograph shows two synaptic densities with clustering of synaptic vesicles in correspondence active zones at the giant synapse (arrows **Figure 3**).

In general, synapses are local of communication where the neurons pass signals through their axons to postsynaptic target (dendrites, axon or cell body of another neuron, muscle cells, or glandular cells). There are two types of synapses (electrical and chemical) that differ in structure and function. The neurons that communicate through electrical synapses outlets are connected by gap junctions, through which the electrical impulse signals are passed directly from pre- to postsynaptic terminals with

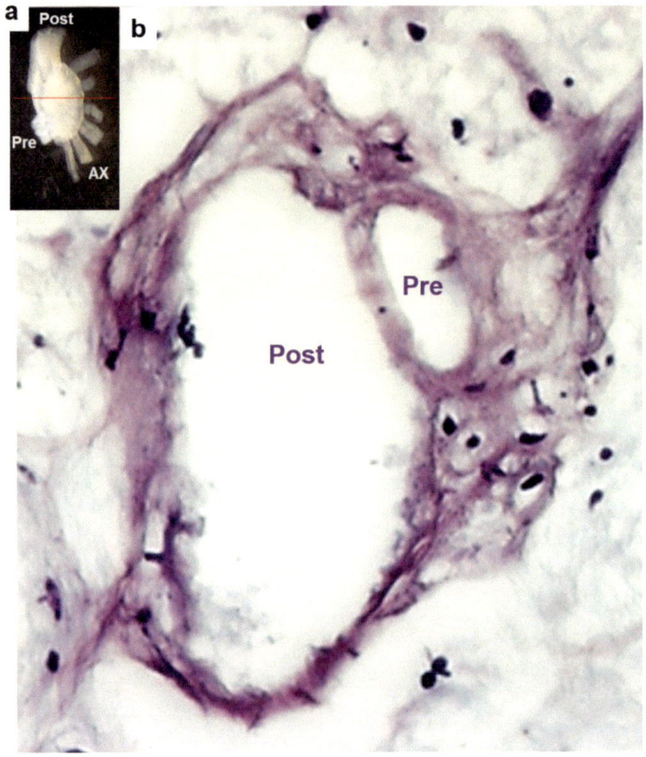

Figure 2.
The giant synapse. a) Stellate ganglion visualized in seawater show presynaptic axon (pre); postsynaptic axon (post) and giant nerve fibers (Ax). The horizontal (line red) illustrates the cross-sectional region from stellate ganglion at giant synapse. b) Light microscopy of cross-sectional region from stellate ganglion shows synaptic contact region between the presynaptic and postsynaptic terminal at giant synapse visualized by H.E. with 40x magnification.

high speed. On the other hand, chemical synapses contain the synaptic vesicles at the presynaptic terminal, which carry specific neurotransmitters and have ion channels in the plasma membrane. What differs between chemical and electrical synapses by electrophysiology approach is their impulse speed with a delay feature around 0.5 ms between them, respectively.

Each synaptic vesicles (SV) consists of an apparatus with hundreds of specific proteins to produce fusion of their membranes with the presynaptic membrane and secrete the neurotransmitters at the synapses. It is integrated by corresponding area of neuron, which contains a part of the postsynaptic density (PSD) with ion channel receptors at the postsynaptic membrane for neurotransmitters [10, 15].

The size of synaptic vesicles is variable and dependent of neurotransmitter type [16]. In general, there are two types of vesicles: electron-dense center vesicle and electron-lucent center vesicle. Electron-dense vesicles are subdivided into two types: containing catecholamines (80 nm) and, large synaptic vesicles that contain neuropeptides (200 nm). On the other hand, electron-lucent vesicles have 50 nm of diameter and been carried out with acetylcholine, glycine, GABA, or glutamate. These vesicles are accumulated close at the active zone with 0.5 mm of distance from the plasma membrane.

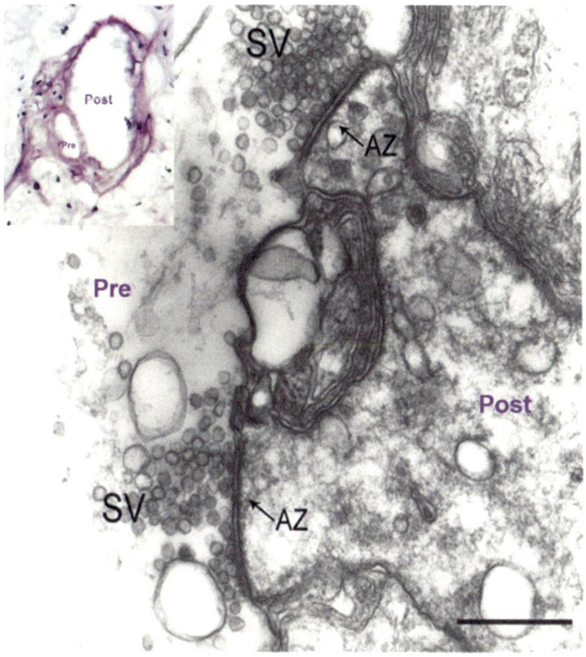

Figure 3.
Ultrastructure of the giant synapse. Electron micrographs of the giant synapse showing clustering of synaptic vesicles (SV) and active zones (AZ). The insert left shows giant synapse with presynaptic and postsynaptic terminal visualized by H.E with 40x magnification. Scale bar represent 0.5 microns (courtesy of Dr. Jorge Moreira-FMRP).

The membrane proteins (SV) are synthesized in the endoplasmic reticulum granular (REG) and carried through vesicles of the Golgi complex to the presynaptic terminal. The motor proteins (kinesin and dynein) make the transport through microtubules [7] and myosin proteins [17–19] through actin filaments [20]. The membrane proteins (SV) probably are selected in the primary endosome, which give rise to the synaptic vesicle that to be filled with neurotransmitters.

In summary, when an action potential reaches in the presynaptic terminal least vesicles fuse with specify region at the presynaptic membrane. The action potential in the presynaptic terminal is a very fast process, which have voltage-operated channels allowing rapid and transient entry of calcium (Ca^{2+}) that interacts with several group of vesicular proteins and membrane protein into presynaptic terminal [7, 21, 22]. However, are many proteins involved with endocytosis and exocytosis process of synaptic vesicles.

The calcium triggers fusion of synaptic vesicle with the presynaptic membrane, whereas the central protein involved in fusion of synaptic vesicles is Synaptotagmin protein, which is defined such a calcium sensor due to its C2A domain. The C2A domain through its interaction with calcium undergoes a conformational change, causing it to fuse phospholipids from vesicle and presynaptic membranes. On the other hand, the C2B domain of Synaptotagmin is involved with recycling of synaptic vesicles [23–25]. Finally, electrophysiology and biochemical approaches of synaptic events have been obtained from the squid nervous system studies, in which specific antibodies and homologous proteins were used for knowledge of synaptic events [10, 11, 15, 26–28], and also more recently, genetic approach was showed a knockout of the squid pigmentation gene [29]. This method demonstrated efficient gene knockout in the squid *Doryteuthis pealeii* using CRISPR-Cas9 and should be readily adopted by other research groups because this method does not require specialized equipment and squid are available worldwide.

4. Immunohistochemistry and immunofluorescence studies: squid optic lobe and synaptosome

The complexity of subcellular domains in neurons and their distances of nucleus demand a spatial and temporal control of protein synthesis. We have identified a novel member of hnRNP A/B type, of 65 kDa, in the presynaptic terminal of squid neuron [30–32]. Squid p65 was phylogenetically conserved hnRNP type A/B protein in mammals [33]. In this scenario, these hnRNPs have emerged as major components of mechanisms for the local protein synthesis and synaptic plasticity.

To assess their presynaptic terminal location in squid photoreceptors neurons, the immunohistochemistry of slices from optic lobe was incubated with the anti-synaptic vesicle glycoprotein 2A (α-SV2) antibody and developed by peroxidase-DAB (see in method). The α-SV2 antibody recognizes the corresponding bands in the outer plexiform layer (**Figure 4a**), which is a synaptic connection region [34]. This image was similar to those previously obtained with the Synaptotagmin antibody [31]. These data showed an anatomy is highly complex with outer cortical layers and a central medulla from squid optic lobe [35–37].

To further indicate the subcellular localization of hnRNPs is involved in presynaptic terminal localization in squid photoreceptors neurons, the synaptosomes isolated from optic lobes were double probed with α-SV2 antibody and anti-squid ribonucleoprotein motif 2 (α-sqRNP2) antibody raised in rabbits [30]. Immunofluorescence microscopy of synaptosomes showed intense granular staining with both antibodies frequently close to the plasma membrane, suggesting a spatial relationship between both proteins to clustering synaptic vesicle at the presynaptic terminal (**Figure 4b**).

In fact, hnRNP protein shuttles mature mRNA from nucleus to the cytoplasm and are also involved in packaging mRNAs into cytoplasmic granule transport, which have been more clearly evidenced in dendrite cells. However, the exact function of hnRNPs in the presynaptic terminal has yet to be clarified [31, 38].

5. hnRNP proteins and degenerative diseases

Several cellular compartments not enclosed by membranes are called ribonucleoprotein granules, due to the high concentration of proteins and mRNAs (mRNPs). For example, mRNPs can be found in the nucleus in Cajal bodies, paraspeckles, speckles, etc., but they can also be found in the cytoplasm, such as stress granules and processing bodies (Pbodies).

Stress granules are cytoplasmic complexes made up of proteins and RNA, found in most cell types in culture (from yeast to humans), and are formed under specific conditions of cellular stress [39]. *In vitro* experiments with different conditions can induce the formation of stress granules such as lack of nutrients, heating, protein complex and protein degradation inhibitors (proteasome), genotoxic drugs (such as UV radiation), and drugs that cause oxidative stress (sodium arsenite) or osmotic

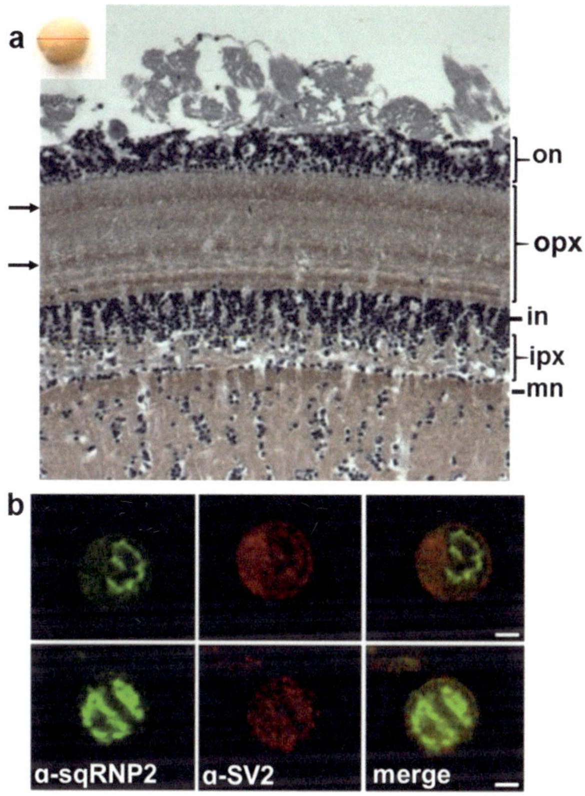

Figure 4.
Immunolocalization of presynaptic terminal in the optic lobe "chickpeas-like." a) Immunohistochemistry of the 10 nm slice through the squid optic lobe labeled with anti-vesicle protein 2 antibody (a-SV2) and secondary antibody by the peroxidase-DAB (method described by [31]). The arrows indicate the immunopositive bands for both antibodies in the outer plexiform layer (opx). The morphological layers of the optic lobe cortex are indicated to the right: Outer nuclear (on), outer plexiform (opx), inner nuclear (in), inner plexiform (ipx), and mononuclear (mn) layers with optic nerve terminals at the outer plexiform layer (opx) from optic lobe cortex. Scale bars 100 µm. b) Confocal images of two representative synaptosomes that were double immunolabeled with anti-sqRNP2 antibody (a-sqRNP2, green) and anti-vesicle protein 2 antibody (a-SV2, red). The merged images show yellow where overlap occurs. Scale bars 2 µm.

agent (sorbitol) [39, 40]. Many studies showed an association of mRNPs to neurodegenerative diseases [41–45].

Of course, stress granules are generated as a cellular response to a physiologically unfavorable environment, and their prevalence in neurological disorders suggests that their formation in affected neurons is, at least initially, a cytoprotective response to disease-associated stress. However, the persistence of stress granules can contribute to the development of several degenerative diseases, such as amyotrophic lateral sclerosis (ALS), frontotemporal lobar degeneration (FTLD), and some myopathies and neurodegenerative diseases [46].

The mutations in RNA-binding proteins appear to increase the propensity of these proteins to aggregate and form stress granules. For example, diseases linked to mutations promote aggregation in the proteins such as TDP-43 (TAR DNA-binding protein 43) and FUS (Fused in Sarcoma) [43–45, 47–49].

In previous studies [30, 50] showed molecular and biochemical evidence that p65 is a dimer resistant to SDS treatment, composed of two protein subunits of the hnRNP A/B type with molecular weight around 37 kDa, and this propensity of these proteins to aggregate and form stress granules involves endogenous modification factors. Nevertheless, it did not clear show how such endogenous factors could act to produce alterations in hnRNP A/B-like protein that induces dimerization. Immunohistochemical studies demonstrate the presence of p65 in presynaptic nerve terminals and its propensity to oligomerize led us to further investigate their cellular and molecular properties in presynaptic nerve terminals [50].

In conclusion, based on these points presented here, we suggest that hnRNP A/B protein could be a link between local RNA processing and synaptic function at the presynaptic terminal. Understanding this can bring insights into evolution of several neurodegenerative diseases and verify if they resemble the function performed in vertebrates.

This brief summary has shown that the cephalopods have structure's power that served in comparative studies and useful alternative to invertebrate experimental research that, in general, is applicable to mammalian systems. However, are few studies with biochemical and molecular approach, which could lead to a better understanding of their physiological functions.

6. Materials and methods

6.1 Animals and tissue preparation

The optic lobes were dissected from freshly killed *D. pealei* obtained from the Marine Biological Laboratory in Woods Hole or from *D. plei* obtained from the Centro de Biologia Marinha-CEBIMar, University of São Paulo, São Sebastião, Brazil. For immunohistochemistry and immunofluorescence procedures freshly dissected optic lobes are from *D. ssp* [31]. The synaptosomes (isolated nerve terminals from photoreceptor cells) were prepared from tissue according to Pekkurnaz et al. [51] with slight modifications. Briefly, optic lobes were quickly dissected from squid onto ice-cold Petri dishes and weighed. Each g of tissue was homogenized in 5 ml of ice-cold homogenization buffer (HB) (1.0 M sucrose in 20 mM Tris-HCl, pH 7.4) in a Wheaton glass homogenizer with a loose-fitting pestle, by 10–15 gentle strokes. The homogenate was spun at 1000xg for 11 min at 4 °C and then spun at 13,000xg for 45 min. The floating synaptosome layer was carefully decanted into a small Petri dish, gently washed in HB and resuspended in 0.5 ml of HB.

6.2 Antibodies

Anti-squid ribonucleoprotein motif 2 (α-sqRNP2) antibody was raised in rabbits. The α-sqRNP2 antibody raised in rabbits against the synthetic peptide CLFIGGLSYDTNEDTIK corresponds to an internal sequence determined by mass spectrometry from tissue-purified p65 [30]. The rabbit serum after inoculation was purified on a HiTrap Recombinant Protein A column (GE Health Science, Chalfont St.Giles, UK) by Fast protein liquid chromatography (ÄKTAFPLC system). The monoclonal anti-synaptic vesicle glycoprotein 2A (α-SV2) antibody (64,051, Invitrogen, Carlsbad, CA) was raised in mouse and secondary antibodies conjugated to Alexa 488 for immunofluorescence from Molecular Probes (Invitrogen, Carlsbad, CA).

6.3 Ultrastructure

The stellate ganglion was removed from squid mantle on the seawater, fixed by immersion in 2% formaldehyde plus 2% glutaraldehyde in buffered calcium-free seawater, postfixed in osmium tetroxide, stained with uranium acetate, dehydrated, and embedded in Araldite plastic CY212 (EMS). Ultra-thin sections in carbon-coated single-slot grids were contrasted with uranyl acetate and lead citrate. Electron micrographs were taken at an initial magnification of x14,000 and photographically enlarged to a magnification of x35,000.

6.4 Immunohistochemistry

Fixed, 1-mm transversal slices of optic lobes were included in Paraplast (Oxford Labwase, St. Louis, MO, USA) following the manufacturer's instructions. Microtome slices of 10 µm were cut, transferred to glass slides, de-parafinized, and rehydrated by standard procedures. Slices were incubated in PBS pH 7.4 containing 0.1 M glycine for 30 min at 4°C to block aldehyde groups and then washed three times for 10 min in PBS. They were then incubated in the dark at room temperature for 30 min in methanol containing 0.9% hydrogen peroxide solution to inhibit endogenous peroxidase activity, followed by washing in PBS. The samples were permeabilized and blocked by incubation in PBS containing 1% Triton X-100, 3% BSA, and 0.5% sheep serum and then incubated for 1 h with primary antibodies in PBS containing 0.1% Triton X-100, 3% BSA, and 0.5% sheep serum. After washing in PBS containing 0.1% Triton X-100, the slices were incubated for 1 h with secondary antibodies conjugated to horse radish peroxidase (KPL, Gaithersburg, MD, USA) diluted 1:400 in PBS containing 0.1% Triton X-100, 3% BSA, and 0.5% sheep serum and developed using 3,3-diaminobenzidina (DAB) as substrate.

6.5 Immunofluorescence

Synaptosomes in suspension were fixed in 1% paraformaldehyde for 6 hr. at room temperature, adhered to glass microscope slides by incubation for 1 hr. After gentle washing with PBS, slides were incubated for 30 min in 0.1 M glycine, 0.3% Triton X-100 in PBS, pH 7.4, and washed and blocked in 1 mg/ml BSA, 1% goat serum, and 1% Triton X-100 for 1 hr. at room temperature. The slides were washed with PBS containing 0.3% Triton X-100 and incubated with primary antibody in PBS containing 1 mg/ml BSA, 1% goat serum, and 0.3% Triton X-100 for 2 hrs. at room temperature. The slides were washed in PBS and incubated with appropriate secondary antibody for 1 hr. and washed again. The slides were mounted in Fluoromount G (EMS) diluted 2:1 in PBS and examined on a Zeiss 510 confocal microscope.

Acknowledgements

Dr. Gabriel Sarti Lopes and Dr. Jorge E. Moreira of University of São Paulo, FMRP/USP and Dra. Janaina Brusco from University of British Columbia, Can. Financial support from Fundação de Amparo à Pesquisa do Estado de São Paulo (FAPESP), and Conselho Nacional de Desenvolvimento Científico e Tecnológico (CNPq) are acknowledged. Special thanks to Dr. Roy E. Larson of University of São Paulo, FMRP/USP (past advisor). Infrastructure support from Marine Biology Center at University of São Paulo (CEBIMar-USP) and Marine Biological Laboratory, Woods Hole-US. Special thanks to Patricia Horta, PhD, IFSP, that revised this chapter.

Conflict of interest

The author declares that there is no conflict of interests regarding the publication of this chapter.

Author details

Diego Torrecillas Paula Lico
University of São Paulo, SP State, São Paulo, Brazil

*Address all correspondence to: ditplico@gmail.com

References

[1] Young JZ. Structure of nerve fibres in sepia. Journal of Physiology Land. 1935;**83**:27P-28P

[2] Roper CF, Voss GL. Guidelines for taxonomic descriptions of cephalopod species. Memoirs. National Museum of Victoria. 1983;**44**:49-63

[3] Bullock TH. Comparative neuroethology of startle, rapid escape, and giant fibre-mediated responses. In: Eaton RC, editor. Neural Mechanisms of Start I Behavior. New York and London: Plenum Press; 1984. pp. 1-13

[4] Mackie GO. Giant axons and the control of jetting in the squid *Loligo* and the jellyfish *Aglantha*. Canadian Journal of Zoology. 1990;**68**:799-805

[5] Gilly WF, Hopkins B, Mackie GO. Development of giant motor axons and neural control of escape responses in squid embryos and hatchlings. Biology I Bulletin. 1991;**180**:209-220

[6] Roper CFE, Ross KJ. The giant squid. Science. 1982;**246**:96-105

[7] Vale RD, Reese TS, Sheetz MP. Identification of a novel force-generating protein kinesin involved in microtubule-based motility. Cell. 1985;**42**:39-50

[8] Katz B, Miledi R. Membrane noise produced by acetylcholine. Nature. 1970;**226**:962-963

[9] Llinás R, Sugimori M, Simon SM. Transmission by presynaptic spike-like depolarization in the squid giant synapse. Proceedings of the National Academy of Sciences of the United States of America. 1982;**79**:2415-2419

[10] Fukuda M, Moreira JE, Lewis FMT, Sugimori M, Niinobe M, Mikoshiba K, et al. Role of the C2b domain of synaptogamin in transmitter release as determined by specific antibody injection into the squid giant synapse preterminal. Proceedings of the National Academy of Sciences USA. 1995;**92**:10703-10707

[11] Sugimori M, Tong C, Fukuda M, Moreira JE, Kojima T, Mikoshiba K, et al. Presynaptic injection of syntaxin-specific antibodies block transmission in the squid giant synapse. Neuroscience. 1998;**86**:39-51

[12] Gioio AE, Lavina ZS, Jurkovicova D, Zhang H, Eyman M, Giuditta A, et al. Nerve terminals of squid photoreceptor neurons contain a heterogeneous population of mRNAs and translate a transfected reporter mRNA. The European Journal of Neuroscience. 2004;**20**:865-872

[13] Giuditta A, Kaplan BB, van Minnen J, Alvarez J, Koenig E. Axonal and presynaptic protein synthesis: New insights into the biology of the neuron. Trends in Neurosciences. 2002;**25**:400-404

[14] Martin KC, Casadio A, Zhu H, Yaping E, Rose JC, Chen M, et al. Synapse-specific, long-term facilitation of aplysia sensory to motor synapses: A function for local protein synthesis in memory storage. Cell. 1997;**91**:927-938

[15] Mikoshiba K, Fukuda M, Moreira JE, Lewis FMT, Sugimori M, Niinobe M, et al. Role of the C2b of synaptogmin in vesicular release and recycling as determined by specific antibody injection into the squid giant synapse preterminal. Proceedings of the National Academy of Sciences USA. 1995;**92**:10708-10712

[16] Burns ME, Augustine GJ. Synaptic structure and function: Dynamic organization yields architectural precision. Cell. 1995;**83**:187-194

[17] Calliari A, Sotelo-Silveira J, Costa MC, Nogueira J, Cameron LC, Kun A, et al. Myosin Va is locally synthesized following nerve injury. Cell Motility and the Cytoskeleton. 2002;**51**:169-176

[18] Ohashi S, Koike K, Omori A, Ichinose S, Ohara S, Kobayashi S, et al. Identification of mRNA/protein (mRNP) complexes containing Puralpha, mStaufen, fragile X protein, and myosin Va and their association with rough endoplasmic reticulum equipped with a kinesin motor. The Journal of Biological Chemistry. 2002;**277**:37804-37810

[19] Sotelo-Silveira JR, Calliari A, Cardenas M, Koenig E, Sotelo JR. Myosin Va and kinesin II motor proteins are concentrated in ribosomal domains (periaxoplasmic ribosomal plaques) of myelinated axons. Journal of Neurobiology. 2004;**60**:187-196

[20] Bearer EL, Debirgis JA, Boduer RA, Aw K, Reese TS. Evidence for miosin motors on organelles in squid axoplasm. Proceedings of the National Academy of Sciences USA. 1993;**90**:11252-11256

[21] Edwards RH. The transport of neurotransmitters into synaptic vesicles. Current Opinion in Neurobiology. 1992;**2**:586-594

[22] Régnier-Vigouroux A, Tooze AS, Huttner WB. Newly synthesized synaptophysin is transported to synaptic-like microvesicles via constitutive secretory vesicles and the plasma membrane. The EMBO Journal. 1991;**10**:3589-3601

[23] Betz WJ, Bewick GS. Optical monitoring of neurotransmitter release and synaptic vesicle recycling at the frog neuromuscular junction. Journal of Physiology (London). 1993;**460**:287-309

[24] Hata Y, Slaughter CA, Sudhof TC. Synaptic vesicle fusion complex contains unc-18 homologue bound to syntaxin. Nature. 1993;**366**:347-351

[25] Ryan TA, Smith SJ. Vesicle pool mobilization during action potential firing at hippocampal synapses. Neuron. 1995;**14**:983-989

[26] Gainer H, Galdlant PE, Gould R, Pant HC. Biochemistry and metabolism of the squid Giant axon. Current Topics in Membranes and Transport. 1984;**22**:57-90

[27] Llinás RR, Sugimori M, Lang EJ, Morita M, Fukuda M, Niinobe M, et al. The inositol high-polyphosphate series block synaptic transmission by preventing vesicular fusion: A squid giant synapse. Proceedings of the National Academy of Sciences USA. 1994;**91**:12990-12993

[28] Marsal J, Ruiz-Montacell B, Blasi J, Moreira JE, Contreras D, Sugimori M, et al. Block of transmitter release by botulinium C1 action on syntaxin at the squid giant synapse. Proceedings of the National Academy of Sciences USA. 1997;**94**:14871-14876

[29] Karen C, Diaz JF, Quiroz KM, Koenig NA, Albertin CB, Rosenthal JJC. Highly efficient knockout of a squid pigmentation gene. Current Biology. 2020;**30**:3484-3490

[30] Lico DT, Lopes GS, Brusco J, Rosa JC, Gould RM, De Giorgis JA, et al. A novel SDS-stable dimer of a heterogeneous nuclear ribonucleoprotein at presynaptic terminals of squid neurons. Neuroscience. 2015;**300**:381-392

[31] Lico DTP, Rosa JC, DeGiorgis JA, deVasconcelos EJR, Casaletti L, Tauhata SBF, et al. A novel 65 kDa RNA-binding protein in squid presynaptic terminals. Neuroscience. 2010;**166**:73-83

[32] Lopes GS, Brusco J, Rosa JC, Larson RE, DTP L. Selectively RNA

interaction by a hnRNPA/B-like protein at presynaptic terminal of squid neuron. Invertebrate Neuroscience. 2020;**20**:14

[33] Lopes GS, Lico DTP, Rocha RS, Oliveira RR, Sebollela AS, Paco-Larson ML, et al. A phylogenetically conserved hnRNP type A/B protein from squid brain. Neuroscience Letters. 2019;**696**:219-224

[34] Haghighat N, Cohen RS, Pappas GD. Fine structure of squid (*Loligo pealei*) optic lobe synapses. Neuroscience. 1984;**13**:527-546

[35] Budelmann BU. Cephalopod sense organs, nerves and the brain: Adaptations for high performance and life style. Marine and Freshwater Behaviour and Physiology. 1994;**25**:13-33

[36] Young JZ. The Anatomy of the Nervous System of Octopus vulgaris. Oxford: Clarendon Press; 1971

[37] Young JZ. The central nervous system of Loligo. I. the optic lobe. Philosophical Transactions of Royal Society of London B. 1974;**267**:263-302

[38] Gabriel LS, Janaina B, Jose RC, Roy LE, Diego LTP. Selectively RNA interaction by a hnRNPA/B-like protein at presynaptic terminal of squid neuron. Invertebrate Neuroscience. 2020;**20**:1-14

[39] Dimasi P et al. Modulation of p-eIF2α cellular levels and stress granule assembly/disassembly by trehalose. Scientific Reports. 2017;**7**:44088

[40] Mahboubi H, Stochaj U. Cytoplasmic stress granules: Dynamic modulators of cell signaling and disease. Biochimica et Biophysica Acta - Molecular Basis of Disease. 2017;**1863**:884-895

[41] Aulas A, Vande Velde C. Alterations in stress granule dynamics driven by TDP-43 and FUS: A link to pathological inclusions in ALS? Frontiers in Cellular Neuroscience. 2015;**9**:423

[42] Heraviab YB, Van Broeckhovenab C, der Zee J. Stress granule mediated protein aggregation and underlying gene defects in the FTD-ALS spectrum. Neurobiology of Disease. 2020;**134**:104639

[43] Polymenidou M, Cleveland DW. Biological spectrum of amyotrophic lateral sclerosis prions. Cold Spring Harbor Perspectives in Medicine. 2017;**7**:a024133

[44] Ramaswami M, Taylor JP, Parker R. Altered ribostasis: RNA-protein granules in neurodegenerative disorders. Cell. 2013;**154**:727-736

[45] Zhang K, Daigle JG, Cunningham KM, Coyne AN, Ruan K, Grima JC, et al. Stress granule assembly disrupts nucleocytoplasmic transport. Cell. 2018;**173**:958-971.e917

[46] Li Y et al. RBM45 homo-oligomerization mediates association with ALS-linked proteins and stress granules. Scientific Reports. 2015;**5**:14262

[47] Ash PEA et al. Pathological stress granules in Alzheimer's disease. Brain Research. 2014;**1584**:52-58

[48] Kim HJ, Kim NC, Wang Y-D, Scarborough EA, Moore J, et al. Mutations in prion-like domains in hnRNPA2B1 and hnRNPA1 cause multisystem proteinopathy and ALS. Nature. 2013;**495**:467-473

[49] Wolozin B. Regulated protein aggregation: Stress granules and neurodegeneration. Molecular Neurodegeneration. 2012;7(1):56

[50] Gabriel S. Lopes and Lico DT P. Biochemical and subcellular characterization of a squid hnRNPA/B-like protein in osmotic stress activated

cells reflects molecular properties conserved in this protein family. Molecular Biology Reports. 2022. DOI: 10.1007/s11033-022-07260-0

[51] Pekkurnaz G, Fera A, Zimmerberg-Helms J, DeGiorgis JA, Bezrukov L, Blank PS, et al. Isolation and ultrastructural characterization of squid synaptic vesicles. Biology Bulletin. 2011;**220**:89-96

Section 4

Cardiovascular Research in Large Animals

Chapter 11

Large Animal Models in Cardiovascular Research

Hiroaki Osada, Kozue Murata and Hidetoshi Masumoto

Abstract

Studies of not only preclinical cardiovascular research but also those of life science, medical, and pharmacological fields commonly utilize small animal models. However, for the advancement of cardiovascular medicine, researches using large animal models are important step for preclinical validation of therapeutic efficacy and safety by virtue of having models with a body and heart size comparable with that of a human, providing clinically relevant experiments without the concern of over- or under-estimating therapeutic effects and risks. In particular, pigs are considered as a suitable animal model for research in cardiovascular medicine because of the similarities in physiology, metabolism, genomics, and proteomics to those in humans. Another advantage of pigs is the availability of various heart disease models such as myocardial infarction and genetically established cardiomyopathy. The present review updates the contributions of large animal model-based research to the development of cardiovascular medicine, especially focusing on the utility of pig models.

Keywords: large animal models, cardiovascular research, translational research, pig models, disease models

1. Introduction

Studies of not only preclinical cardiovascular research but also those of life science, medical, and pharmacological fields commonly utilize small animal models such as rodents. However, the translation of the rodent-based results to clinical trials does not always provide relevant results in humans possibly due to anatomical differences between humans and small animals, or variations in physiological characteristics and mechanisms of the disease development [1–3]. To confirm safety and efficacy in clinical studies, the transition from small-to-large animal studies, which comprise anatomical, biological, and physiological features similar to humans, is anticipated. Therefore, the selection of animal species and preparation of suitable disease models are crucial to obtain clinically relevant results leading to a better translation to human clinical practices [4, 5].

Among traditionally used large animal models in research like non-human primates, horses, bovines, sheep, goats, dogs, cats, and pigs, the pig model is considered to be a desirable experimental model because of its similarity to humans in terms of body and heart size to humans, enabling the researcher to prepare clinically relevant disease models such as a myocardial infarction model [6]. Other advantages of the pig model are its similarities in physiology, metabolism, genomics, and proteomics to humans [7–10]. Genetically modified pig disease models, such as the genetic cardiomyopathy model, have also been developed [11]. The current review updates the contributions of large animal models for research of cardiovascular medicine, especially focusing on the utility of pig models.

2. Advantages of large animal models for cardiovascular research

2.1 Clinical relevance by virtue of the proximity in size to humans

To develop therapeutic materials and procedures in cardiovascular medicine, preclinical validation of therapeutic efficacy and safety of medical materials using large animal models is an important step considering the comparable body and heart size with those in humans, which provides clinically relevant experimental procedures (**Figure 1**).

Since Gibbon first described cardiac surgery using cardiopulmonary bypass more than a half century ago [12], it is no overstatement to say that the history of cardiac surgery is the history of cardiopulmonary bypass development. Large animal models such as sheep and baboons have been used for the development of cardiopulmonary bypass and perioperative management, including anesthesia management models [13–17]. In the recent development of left ventricular assist devices (LVADs) for severe heart failure, large animal models such as bovine, dog, goat, pig, and sheep have been used. The device itself and cannula design, the surgical technique, performance, and the integration within the cardiovascular system must translate from these large animals to human patients [18]. Bovines, such as calves, are considered the most useful large animal model for this study [19].

On the other hand, Stephenson et al. reported the feasibility of the usage of Holstein calves in developing a robotically assisted microsurgical system to perform coronary artery anastomoses [20]. In another review, studies on the pathophysiology

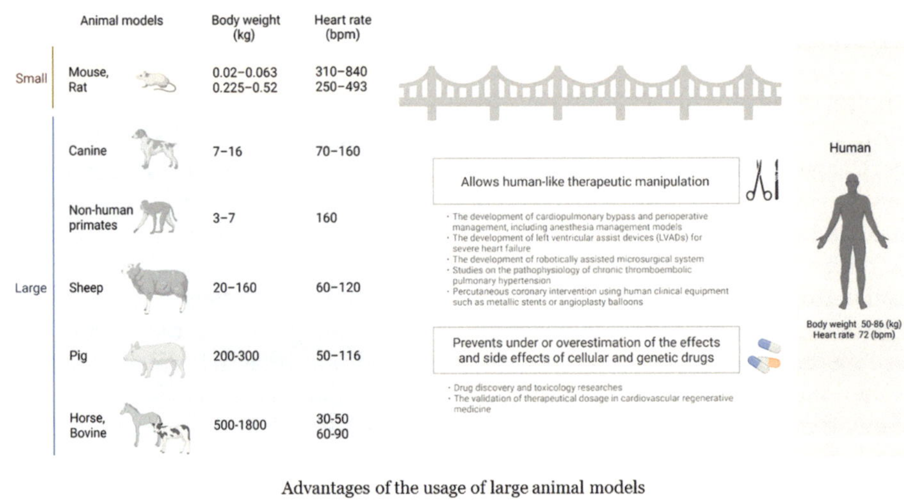

Figure 1.
Advantages of the usage of large animal models.

of chronic thromboembolic pulmonary hypertension using large animal models such as dogs and pigs using either indwelling or Swan Ganz catheters are summarized [21]. An important translational feature of pig models is the possibility of percutaneous coronary intervention using human clinical equipment, and the procedures using metallic stents or angioplasty balloons [22, 23]. These previous reports indicate the importance of using large animal models with similar cardiovascular system sizes to that of humans, enabling human-like experiments.

Additionally, in primary screening tests of drug discovery and toxicology studies, rodents such as mice and rats are mainly used [5]. However, the risk of under- or overestimation of the therapeutic efficacy or side effects remains in studies using animal models where the size of the body and the organs differ so much from humans. Recently, large animals are increasingly taking place as an alternative to rodents [9, 10]. Especially, mini-pigs have been largely utilized as they are easier to handle and suitable for drug discovery and toxicology researches. In addition to their anatomical and physiological similarities to humans, mini-pigs can be used for all routes of drug administration, such as the dietary, continuous intravenous infusion, dermal, or inhalation routes. Furthermore, compared to other laboratory animals, mini-pigs have a much closer metabolism of chemicals to humans [24–26].

Large animal models have been recently introduced not only in pharmaceutical toxicology evaluations but also in cardiovascular regenerative medicine using cell-free materials such as exosomes, microRNAs, proteins such as growth factors, and extracellular matrix components [27]. Therefore, it would be possible that the validation of therapeutical dosage in cardiovascular regenerative medicine would also be tested in preclinical efficacy and safety tests using large animal models [28].

2.2 Advantage of pigs as a large animal model

Pigs are considered a suitable model for cardiovascular research because of the similarities in anatomy, physiology, metabolism, genomics, and proteomics to those in humans (**Figure 2**). Compared with other animal models, pigs acquire early sexual maturity, sizeable litter size, and have a quick reproduction time. They also breed year-round, which makes them highly suitable for biomedical research programs [29]. On the other hand, like other animals, there is moderate genetic variation between breeds (such as the human population) and within breeds that makes variations in the occurrence of abiogenetic diseases [30].

There are several advantages of pigs as a model animal for research in cardiovascular medicine as listed below:

i. The heart size of pigs and its relative weight to body weight is similar to those of the human heart, therefore similar to human patients. In this context, multiple and longitudinal measurements using imaging modalities (echocardiography, computed tomography, magnetic resonance imaging, etc.) and access to biopsies and postmortem samples are possible.

ii. Resemblance to human cardiac physiology, such as ventricular performance and electrophysiology: there is a functional equivalence of various diseases in humans and pigs.

iii. Pigs have negligible collateral circulation, so each coronary artery supplies a specific cardiac region, unlike other laboratory animals [5, 31, 32].

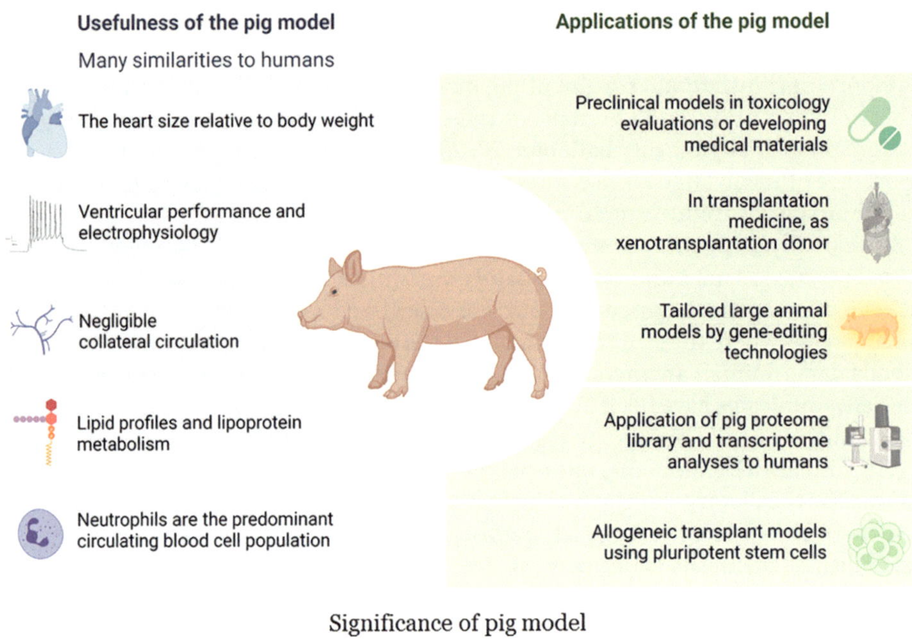

Figure 2.
Significance of the pig model.

Furthermore, the porcine cardiovascular system shares many similarities with those of humans, not only in the anatomical structure but also in the lipid profiles and lipoprotein metabolism, and is known to develop spontaneous lesions in the vasculature and cardiac valves [33]. Likewise, pigs show greater similarity to humans as neutrophils are also the predominant circulating blood cell population [34].

Based on these advantages, pig models are widely used in preclinical models in toxicology evaluations or developing medical materials, taking advantage of their anatomical characteristics. Their natural characteristics have also been widely used in the research of aortic valve stenosis, vascular calcification, and atherosclerosis [35–37]. In transplantation medicine, pigs have also been proposed as xenotransplantation donors. Due to the donor shortage, these procedures might enable the future xenotransplantation of porcine organs into humans as the main approach for transplantation medicine [38, 39].

Large animal models are also advantageous allowing much more precise disease model preparations compared to those in small animal models, which enables to create predictable injury sizes at a preferred region of the myocardium [40]. In this context, pig modes are largely used to create myocardial infarction models for stem-cell-based regenerative medicine research [6, 41]. Munz et al. reported a surgical myocardial infarction through permanent coronary ligation that provided a reproducible and standardized pig myocardial infarction model. They showed that the optimal occlusion site in terms of morbidity, mortality, and lesion extent was the midpoint of the left anterior descending artery [31]. On the other hand, ameroid constrictors have been used to create a gradual coronary artery occlusion that might avoid lethal arrhythmia during surgical ischemia induction [42, 43]. Catheter-based coronary occlusion models are reported as well [44, 45].

3. Genetic modification to create disease models

3.1 Genetically modified clinically relevant disease large animal models

Precise and efficient gene-editing technologies enable the generation of tailored large animal models of human diseases that could contribute to the development of new diagnostic tests and therapeutic procedures [35, 46]. Developmental engineering technology has been used to create large animal models. In 1985, Hammer et al. reported genetically engineered livestock animals [47]. In 1997, Petters et al. presented the first transgenic livestock animal disease model, a pig model of retinitis pigmentosa, which expressed a mutated rhodopsin gene [48]. Recent advances in innovative methods, such as intracytoplasmic sperm injection-mediated gene transfer and somatic cell nuclear transfer (SNCT), enabled design-specific animal models, such as "Dolly," a cloned sheep [49]. Since then, many genetically engineered models of human disease have been generated through large animal models. By integrating SNCT technology and recently developed gene-editing platforms, including TALENs and the CRISPR/Cas9 system, even more diverse modifications of the genomes of livestock species will be seen in the future [50–52]. The commonly used SCNT approach allows concurrent production of transgenic animals expressing a marker gene and non-transgenic clone siblings from the same nuclear donor cells. The cloned animals would provide a useful syngeneic transplantation model [53].

3.2 Specific disease models in pigs

The pig genome has been extensively sequenced and gene-editing technology has been applied to multiple pig strains so far [5, 54]. These techniques have been already largely applied to pigs to create a model for several diseases, such as cystic fibrosis, diabetes mellitus, and neuromuscular disorder [50].

Regarding a model for cardiovascular diseases, Matsunari et al. recently established a genetically modified pig cardiomyopathy model in which they knocked out the δ-sarcoglycan (δ-SG) gene (SGCD) of domestic pigs by the combination of efficient de novo gene editing and SCNT. SGCD-/- cloned pigs exhibit systolic dysfunction similar to that found in human dilated cardiomyopathy and are expected to be highly applicable for the exploration of the feasibility, safety, and efficacy of therapeutic strategies, as well as for elucidating the underlying mechanisms of new treatments for genetic cardiomyopathy [11, 53].

Blutke et al. established a comprehensive biobank of long-term diabetic INSC94Y transgenic pigs, a model of mutant INS gene-induced diabetes of youth (MIDY), which is a model of poorly controlled diabetes mellitus. It is designed to help diabetes researchers discover the molecules and mechanisms involved in the long-term complications of the disease [7, 55]. Furthermore, it would be possible to create human-like atherosclerotic disease models using this severe diabetes mellitus model in the future. Klymiuk et al. established a tailored pig model of Duchenne muscular dystrophy (DMD) by deleting DMD exon 52 in male pig cells and showed the similarity of the transcriptome in dystrophin-deficient pigs with patients with DMD [8]. This technology might pave the way to establish a DMD-related cardiomyopathy model.

3.3 Genetic labeling of somatic cells for the investigations of therapeutic mechanisms

Genetically modified animal models with fluorescent marker genes by SCNT are highly useful as they enable a more efficient monitoring method of cell survival and cellular kinetics *in vivo* after cell product transplantation [53, 56]. Matsunari et al. produced transgenic-cloned pigs carrying the humanized Kusabira-Orange (huKO) gene, yielding an orange-red fluorescence in its dimeric form. The clear red fluorescence of the huKO protein is maintained in paraffin-embedded tissue sections. The pigs express fluorescent protein not only in various organs but also in pig stem cells or progenitor cells [57].

In hepatocytes or liver organoid transplantation experiments, donor cells/organoids were derived from transgenic KO-expressing pigs and transplanted KO-negative littermate, which showed the distribution and survival of transplanted materials [58, 59]. These techniques are also used in allograft ligament construction to analyze intrinsic and extrinsic cellular dynamics during graft healing [60]. It would also be applicable in research of cardiac regenerative medicine using stem cells in which the tracing of survived cells after transplantation and the mechanisms of graft and host interaction have been investigated by 3-dimensional (3D) imaging of heart tissue after tissue clearing using light-sheet microscopy [61, 62]. Upon distinguishing recipient and donor cells in transplanted grafts, KO-expressing pigs may become sufficient genetic modification models for the 3D posttransplantation analysis of vascular network formation inside of the graft.

4. Future directions of large animal model-based cardiovascular research

4.1 Pig proteomics and the extrapolation to humans

Recent efforts have been focused on the characterization of experimental animals at the molecular level such as genomics, transcriptomics, and proteomics [35] which revealed the close similarity of proteomics in pigs and humans. Since matrix-assisted laser desorption/ionization mass spectrometry (MALDI-MS) was first reported in the 1980s, the technologies have been successfully used in genome, proteome, metabolome, and clinical diagnostic research [63]. It is useful in qualitative and quantitative analyses of disease biomarkers in various specimens that lead to not only diagnosis but also risk stratification and guidance in the selection of therapeutic modalities [64]. Linscheid et al. recently performed systematic analyses of cardiac proteomes across cardiac chambers in humans, pigs, and four commonly used animal models and identified and quantified approximately 7,000 proteins, comparing them with respect to cardiac function and mechanisms of diseases [65]. Tamiyakul et al. performed a proteome analysis on the myocardium of the DMD pig model that showed an altered abundance of several proteins such as reduction of myosin-6, which is directly involved in muscle contraction [66]. Müller et al. reported a pig cardiac transcriptome analysis. They assembled 15,926 transcripts, stratified them, and validated the results by complementary mass spectrometry [67]. These attempts to analyze the proteome and transcriptome in animal models and even in humans will play an important role in the future of cardiovascular regenerative medicine. The knowledge of novel heart failure biomarkers may allow a more personalized medicine in the future [68].

4.2 Allogeneic transplantation models for cardiovascular regenerative medicine

In pluripotent stem cell-based cardiovascular regenerative medicine, the advantage of induced pluripotent stem cells (iPSCs)over embryonic stem cells (ESCs) is the availability of autologous cells for the treatment. When iPSC products are generated autologously, better engraftment free from the risk of immune rejection after the transplantation of cell products is theoretically anticipated [69]. Human iPSCs are also expected to mitigate immune rejection after cell/tissue transplantation in human leucocyte antigen (HLA)-controlled allogeneic use, which is investigated in various animal allogeneic transplantation models [70, 71]. The allogeneic use of iPSCs is expected to avoid disadvantages of autologous iPSCs transplantation, such as the cost and time required for quality control of each individual cell line [72]. Furthermore, autologous cell products from patients with genetic disorders such as genetic cardiomyopathy may take over its diseased phenotype that would hamper the therapeutic effects of the products.

Medicetty et al. introduced allogeneic bone marrow-derived cell transplantation to a pig myocardial infarction model in which cells are delivered by catheter directly to the coronary artery. They showed a significant positive modulation of left ventricular function and remodeling [73]. Regarding iPSC-based cardiovascular regenerative medicine, Shiba et al. reported an allogeneic transplantation experiment using cynomolgus monkeys (Macaca fascicularis). iPSC-derived cardiomyocytes from major histocompatibility complex (MHC)-homozygous animals were transplanted into MHC-matched monkeys by direct intra-myocardial injection. Transplanted cardiomyocytes showed electrical coupling to the recipient's heart tissue and survived without immune rejection in monkeys treated with clinically relevant doses of immunosuppressants, whereas the transplantation of cardiomyocytes to MHC-mismatched monkeys even treated with immunosuppressants exhibited immune rejection of grafted cardiomyocytes with severe infiltration of T lymphocytes [74]. Kawamura et al. reported a cynomolgus monkey-based allogeneic transplantation experiment using cell sheets prepared from iPSC-derived cardiomyocytes. In the experiments, the monkeys with immunosuppressants could show fair engraftment of iPSC-derived cardiomyocyte sheets regardless of MHC matching, whereas even MHC-matched iPSC-derived cardiomyocyte sheets could not be sufficiently engrafted without immunosuppressants, indicating the requirement of immunosuppressants even in MHC-matched transplantation, which may prevent minor antigen-triggered immune rejection [75]. These results may indicate that the significance of MHC matching would be attenuated in iPSC-based cardiac regenerative therapy [76]. The establishment of a swine leukocyte antigen (SLA)-identified allogeneic transplantation pig model [77] and investigations of histological and molecular mechanisms of immune rejection attributed by cell transplantation would contribute to develop the strategy to avoid immune rejection associated with allogeneic human iPSC therapies as well as therapeutic mechanisms of the allogeneic transplantation.

Additionally, researchers have been struggling to establish pig somatic stem cell lines such as bone marrow-derived stem cells or live progenitor cells using somatic cell cloning technology, which may realize a syngeneic donor-recipient system in pigs [53]. Furthermore, attempts are being made to establish pluripotent stem cells from pigs such as pig iPSCs or ESCs. Xu et al. reported pig iPSCs generated by infecting pig pericytes and embryonic fibroblasts with a retroviral vector encoding Oct4, Sox2, Klf4, and c-Myc. The pig iPSCs could be differentiated into cell derivatives of all three primary germ layers *in vitro* [78]. Chakritbudsabong et al. also reported the generation of pig embryonic fibroblast-derived iPSCs and their differentiation ability into cardiomyocytes [79]. Choi et al. reported the generation of pluripotent pig ESCs derived from *in vitro*-fertilized and parthenogenetic embryos [80]. Although iPSC generation from various animal species has been attempted and criticized [81], it will largely contribute to the autologous/allogeneic transplantation experiments in the future, which may further promote stem cell-based cardiovascular regenerative medicine.

5. Conclusion

The usefulness of large animal models in cardiovascular medicine, especially pigs, was outlined on the basis of literature. Although the advantages and disadvantages of large animals should be further evaluated, there is a possibility that large animal-based approaches may contribute to the investigations in cardiovascular medicine. On the other hand, it is also recognized that there are opinions not to welcome large animal models for research purpose use and accurate regulation is indispensable. The number of animals used should be reduced to a minimum following the three R's principle (to reduce, refine, and replace animal models). Experiments using animals should be optimized and standardized considering their translatability and the welfare of the animals [82].

Acknowledgements

We appreciate Dr. Laura Yuriko González Teshima (Kyoto University) for her critical reading of the manuscript. This study was funded by Japan Agency for Medical Research and Development (AMED) under Grant Number 20bm0404029h0103 (to H.M.)

Conflict of interest

H.O declares that he has no conflict of interest. K.M. declares that she has no conflict of interest. H.M. has received research grants from Japan Agency for Medical Research and Development (AMED).

Author details

Hiroaki Osada[1], Kozue Murata[1,2] and Hidetoshi Masumoto[1,2]*

1 Department of Cardiovascular Surgery, Graduate School of Medicine, Kyoto University, Kyoto, Japan

2 Clinical Translational Research Program, RIKEN Center for Biosystems Dynamics Research, Kobe, Japan

*Address all correspondence to: hidetoshi.masumoto@riken.jp

References

[1] Bracken MB. Why animal studies are often poor predictors of human reactions to exposure. Journal of the Royal Society of Medicine. 2009;**102**:120-122. DOI: 10.1258/jrsm.2008.08k033

[2] Hackam DG, Redelmeier DA. Translation of research evidence from animals to humans. Journal of the American Medical Association. 2006;**296**:1731-1732. DOI: 10.1001/jama.296.14.1731

[3] Lacro RV, Dietz HC, Sleeper LA, Yetman AT, Bradley TJ, Colan SD, et al. Atenolol versus losartan in children and young adults with Marfa's syndrome. The New England Journal of Medicine. 2014;**371**:2061-2071. DOI: 10.1056/NEJMoa1404731

[4] Mukhamedshina Y, Shulman I, Ogurcov S, Kostennikov A, Zakirova E, Akhmetzyanova E, et al. mesenchymal stem cell therapy for spinal cord contusion: A comparative study on small and large animal models. Biomolecules. 2009;**9**:811. DOI: 10.3390/biom9120811

[5] Ribitsch I, Baptista PM, Lange-Consiglio A, Melotti L, Patruno M, Jenner F, et al. Large animal models in regenerative medicine and tissue engineering: To do or not to do. Frontiers in Bioengineering and Biotechnology. 2020;**8**:972. DOI: 10.3389/fbioe.2020.00972

[6] Ishigami M, Masumoto H, Ikuno T, Aoki T, Kawatou M, Minakata K, et al. Human iPS cell-derived cardiac tissue sheets for functional restoration of infarcted porcine hearts. PLoS One. 2018;**13**:e0201650. DOI: 10.1371/journal.pone.0201650

[7] Blutke A, Renner S, Flenkenthaler F, Backman M, Haesner S, Kemter E, et al. The Munich MIDY Pig Biobank – A unique resource for studying organ crosstalk in diabetes. Molecular Metabolism. 2017;**6**:931-940. DOI: 10.1016/j.molmet.2017.06.004

[8] Klymiuk N, Blutke A, Graf A, Krause S, Burkhardt K, Wuensch A, et al. Dystrophin-deficient pigs provide new insights into the hierarchy of physiological derangements of dystrophic muscle. Human Molecular Genetics. 2013;**22**:4368-4382. DOI: 10.1093/hmg/ddt287

[9] Swindle MM, Makin A, Herron AJ, Clubb FJ Jr, Frazier KS. Swine as models in biomedical research and toxicology testing. Veterinary Pathology. 2012;**49**:344-356. DOI: 10.1177/0300985811402846

[10] Colleton C, Brewster D, Chester A, Clarke DO, Heining P, Olaharski A, et al. The use of minipigs for preclinical safety assessment by the pharmaceutical industry: Results of an IQ DruSafe Minipig Survey. Toxicologic Pathology. 2016;**44**:458-466. DOI: 10.1177/0192623315617562

[11] Matsunari H, Honda M, Watanabe M, Fukushima S, Suzuki K, Miyagawa S, et al. Pigs with delta-sarcoglycan deficiency exhibit traits of genetic cardiomyopathy. Laboratory Investigation. 2020;**100**:887-899. DOI: 10.1038/s41374-020-0406-7

[12] Gibbon JH Jr. Application of a mechanical heart and lung apparatus to cardiac surgery. Minnesota Medicine. 1954;**37**:171-185

[13] Scorsin M, Andreas M, Corona S, Guta AC, Aruta P, Badano LP. Novel transcatheter mitral prosthesis designed to preserve physiological

ventricular flow dynamics. The Annals of Thoracic Surgery. 2022;**113**:593-599. DOI: 10.1016/j.athoracsur.2021.03.067

[14] DiVincenti L Jr, Westcott R, Lee C. Sheep (*Ovis aries*) as a model for cardiovascular surgery and management before, during, and after cardiopulmonary bypass. Journal of the American Association for Laboratory Animal Science. 2014;**53**:439-448

[15] Flynn C, Hurtig M, Lamoure E, Cummins E, Roati V, Lowerison M, et al. Modeling and staging of osteoarthritis progression using serial CT imaging and arthroscopy. Cartilage. 2020;**11**:338-347. DOI: 10.1177/1947603518789997

[16] Fletcher JR, McKee A, Anderson R, Watson L. Baboon veno-arterial cardiopulmonary bypass without anticoagulants. Transactions of the American Society of Artificial Internal Organs. 1978;**24**:315-319

[17] Temple LJ, Ritchie HE, Wright JT, Koziell J. Prolonged partial left heart bypass in sheep: Successful use of a new type of pump. Thorax. 1971;**26**:543-550. DOI: 10.1136/thx.26.5.543

[18] Monreal G, Sherwood LC, Sobieski MA, Giridharan GA, Slaughter MS, Koenig SC. Large animal models for left ventricular assist device research and development. ASAIO Journal. 2014;**60**:2-8. DOI: 10.1097/MAT.0000000000000005

[19] Motomura T, Tuzun E, Yamazaki K, Tatsumi E, Benkowski R, Yamazaki S. Preclinical evaluation of the EVAHEART 2 centrifugal left ventricular assist device in bovines. ASAIO Journal. 2019;**65**:845-854. DOI: 10.1097/MAT.0000000000000869

[20] Stephenson ER Jr, Sankholkar S, Ducko CT, Damiano RJ Jr. Successful endoscopic coronary artery bypass grafting: An acute large animal trial. The Journal of Thoracic and Cardiovascular Surgery. 1998;**116**:1071-1073. DOI: 10.1016/S0022-5223(98)70060-1

[21] Stam K, Clauss S, Taverne Y, Merkus D. Chronic thromboembolic pulmonary Hypertension – What have we learned from large animal models. Front Cardiovasc Med. 2021;**8**:574360. DOI: 10.3389/fcvm.2021.574360

[22] Lowe HC, Schwartz RS, Mac Neill BD, Jang IK, Hayase M, Rogers C, et al. The porcine coronary model of in-stent restenosis: Current status in the era of drug-eluting stents. Catheterization and Cardiovascular Interventions. 2003;**60**:515-523. DOI: 10.1002/ccd.10705

[23] Schwartz RS, Murphy JG, Edwards WD, Camrud AR, Vliestra RE, Holmes DR. Restenosis after balloon angioplasty. A practical proliferative model in porcine coronary arteries. Circulation. 1990;**82**:2190-2200. DOI: 10.1161/01.cir.82.6.2190

[24] Forster R, Bode G, Ellegaard L, van der Laan JW. The RETHINK project on minipigs in the toxicity testing of new medicines and chemicals: Conclusions and recommendations. Journal of Pharmacological and Toxicological Methods. 2010;**62**:236-242. DOI: 10.1016/j.vascn.2010.05.008

[25] Svendsen O. The minipig in toxicology. Experimental and Toxicologic Pathology. 2006;**57**:335-339. DOI: 10.1016/j.etp.2006.03.003

[26] Stricker-Krongrad A, Shoemake CR, Pereira ME, Gad SC, Brocksmith D, Bouchard GF. Miniature swine breeds in toxicology and drug safety assessments: What to expect during clinical and pathology evaluations. Toxicologic Pathology. 2016;**44**:421-427. DOI: 10.1177/0192623315613337

[27] Spannbauer A, Mester-Tonczar J, Traxler D, Kastner N, Zlabinger K, Hasimbegovic E, et al. Large animal models of cell-free cardiac regeneration. Biomolecules. 2020;**10**:1392. DOI: 10.3390/biom10101392

[28] Grigorian-Shamagian L, Sanz-Ruiz R, Climent A, Badimon L, Barile L, Bolli R, et al. Insights into therapeutic products, preclinical research models, and clinical trials in cardiac regenerative and reparative medicine: Where are we now and the way ahead. Current opinion paper of the ESC Working Group on Cardiovascular Regenerative and Reparative Medicine. Cardiovascular Research. 2021;**117**:1428-1433. DOI: 10.1093/cvr/cvaa337

[29] Polejaeva IA, Rutigliano HM, Wells KD. Livestock in biomedical research: History, current status and future prospective. Reproduction, Fertility, and Development. 2016;**28**:112-124. DOI: 10.1071/RD15343

[30] Bendixen E, Danielsen M, Larsen K, Bendixen C. Advances in porcine genomics and proteomics – a toolbox for developing the pig as a model organism for molecular biomedical research. Briefings in Functional Genomics. 2010;**9**:208-219. DOI: 10.1093/bfgp/elq004

[31] Munz MR, Faria MA, Monteiro JR, Aguas AP, Amorim MJ. Surgical porcine myocardial infarction model through permanent coronary occlusion. Comparative Medicine. 2011;**61**:445-452

[32] White FC, Roth DM, Bloor CM. The pig as a model for myocardial ischemia and exercise. Laboratory Animal Science. 1986;**36**:351-356

[33] Gerrity RG, Natarajan R, Nadler JL, Kimsey T. Diabetes-induced accelerated atherosclerosis in swine. Diabetes. 2001;**50**:1654-1665. DOI: 10.2337/diabetes.50.7.1654

[34] Meurens F, Summerfield A, Nauwynck H, Saif L, Gerdts V. The pig: A model for human infectious diseases. Trends in Microbiology. 2012;**20**:50-57. DOI: 10.1016/j.tim.2011.11.002

[35] Tsang HG, Rashdan NA, Whitelaw CB, Corcoran BM, Summers KM, MacRae VE. Large animal models of cardiovascular disease. Cell Biochemistry and Function. 2016;**34**:113-132. DOI: 10.1002/cbf.3173

[36] Porras AM, Shanmuganayagam D, Meudt JJ, Krueger CG, Hacker TA, Rahko PS, et al. Development of aortic valve disease in familial hypercholesterolemic swine: Implications for elucidating disease etiology. Journal of the American Heart Association. 2015;**4**:e002254. DOI: 10.1161/JAHA.115.002254

[37] Skold BH, Getty R, Ramsey FK. Spontaneous atherosclerosis in the arterial system of aging swine. American Journal of Veterinary Research. 1966;**27**:257-273

[38] Shu S, Ren J, Song J. Cardiac xenotransplantation: A promising way to treat advanced heart failure. Heart Failure Review. 2022;**27**:71-91. DOI: 10.1007/s10741-020-09989-x

[39] Reichart B, Langin M, Radan J, Mokelke M, Buttgereit I, Ying J, et al. Pig-to-non-human primate heart transplantation: The final step toward clinical xenotransplantation? The Journal of Heart and Lung Transplantation. 2020;**39**:751-757. DOI: 10.1016/j.healun.2020.05.004

[40] Shin HS, Shin HH, Shudo Y. Current status and limitations of myocardial infarction large animal models in cardiovascular translational research.

Frontiers in Bioengineering and Biotechnology. 2021;**9**:673683. DOI: 10.3389/fbioe.2021.673683

[41] Kawamura M, Miyagawa S, Fukushima S, Saito A, Miki K, Ito E, et al. Enhanced survival of transplanted human induced pluripotent stem cell-derived cardiomyocytes by the combination of cell sheets with the pedicled omental flap technique in a porcine heart. Circulation. 2013;**128**:S87-S94. DOI: 10.1161/CIRCULATIONAHA.112.000366

[42] Aboulgheit A, Karbasiafshar C, Zhang Z, Sabra M, Shi G, Tucker A, et al. Lactobacillus plantarum probiotic induces Nrf2-mediated antioxidant signaling and eNOS expression resulting in improvement of myocardial diastolic function. American Journal of Physiology. Heart and Circulatory Physiology. 2021;**321**:H839-H849. DOI: 10.1152/ajpheart.00278.2021

[43] Miyagawa S, Mizoguchi H, Fukushima S, Imanishi Y, Watabe T, Harada A, et al. New regional drug delivery system by direct epicardial placement of slow-release prostacyclin agonist promise therapeutic angiogenesis in a porcine chronic myocardial infarction. Journal of Artificial Organs. 2021;**24**:465-472. DOI: 10.1007/s10047-021-01259-3

[44] Sun S, Jiang Y, Zhen Z, Lai WH, Liao S, Tse HF. Establishing a swine model of post-myocardial infarction heart failure for stem cell treatment. Journal of Visualized Experiments. May 25, 2020;159. DOI: 10.3791/60392

[45] Kadota S, Carey J, Reinecke H, Leggett J, Teichman S, Laflamme MA, et al. Ribonucleotide reductase-mediated increase in dATP improves cardiac performance via myosin activation in a large animal model of heart failure. European Journal of Heart Failure. 2015;**17**:772-781. DOI: 10.1002/ejhf.270

[46] Yao J, Huang J, Zhao J. Genome editing revolutionize the creation of genetically modified pigs for modeling human diseases. Human Genetics. 2016;**135**:1093-1105. DOI: 10.1007/s00439-016-1710-6

[47] Hammer RE, Pursel VG, Rexroad CE Jr, Wall RJ, Bolt DJ, Ebert KM, et al. Production of transgenic rabbits, sheep and pigs by microinjection. Nature. 1985;**315**:680-683. DOI: 10.1038/315680a0

[48] Petters RM, Alexander CA, Wells KD, Collins EB, Sommer JR, Blanton MR, et al. Genetically engineered large animal model for studying cone photoreceptor survival and degeneration in retinitis pigmentosa. Nature Biotechnology. 1997;**15**:965-970. DOI: 10.1038/nbt1097-965

[49] Campbell KH, McWhir J, Ritchie WA, Wilmut I. Sheep cloned by nuclear transfer from a cultured cell line. Nature. 1996;**380**:64-66. DOI: 10.1038/380064a0

[50] Rogers CS. Genetically engineered livestock for biomedical models. Transgenic Research. 2016;**25**:345-359. DOI: 10.1007/s11248-016-9928-6

[51] Yang SH, Cheng PH, Banta H, Piotrowska-Nitsche K, Yang JJ, Cheng EC, et al. Towards a transgenic model of Huntington's disease in a non-human primate. Nature. 2008;**453**:921-924. DOI: 10.1038/nature06975

[52] Jacobsen JC, Bawden CS, Rudiger SR, McLaughlan CJ, Reid SJ, Waldvogel HJ, et al. An ovine transgenic Huntington's disease model. Human Molecular Genetics. 2010;**19**:1873-1882. DOI: 10.1093/hmg/ddq063

[53] Matsunari H, Nagashima H. Application of genetically modified and cloned pigs in translational research. The Journal of Reproduction and Development. 2009;**55**:225-230. DOI: 10.1262/jrd.20164

[54] Rubin CJ, Megens HJ, Martinez Barrio A, Maqbool K, Sayyab S, Schwochow D, et al. Strong signatures of selection in the domestic pig genome. Proceedings of the National Academy of Sciences of the United States of America. 2012;**109**:19529-19536. DOI: 10.1073/pnas.1217149109

[55] Abbott A. Inside the first pig biobank. Nature. 2015;**519**:397-398. DOI: 10.1038/519397a

[56] Hamanaka S, Ooehara J, Morita Y, Ema H, Takahashi S, Miyawaki A, et al. Generation of transgenic mouse line expressing Kusabira Orange throughout body, including erythrocytes, by random segregation of provirus method. Biochemical and Biophysical Research Communications. 2013;**435**:586-591. DOI: 10.1016/j.bbrc.2013.05.017

[57] Matsunari H, Onodera M, Tada N, Mochizuki H, Karasawa S, Haruyama E, et al. Transgenic-cloned pigs systemically expressing red fluorescent protein. Kusabira-Orange. Cloning Stem Cells. 2008;**10**:313-323. DOI: 10.1089/clo.2008.0024

[58] Tsuchida T, Murata S, Hasegawa S, Mikami S, Enosawa S, Hsu HC, et al. Investigation of clinical safety of human iPS cell-derived liver organoid transplantation to infantile patients in porcine model. Cell Transplantation. 2020;**29**. DOI: 10.1177/0963689720964384

[59] Shigeta T, Hsu HC, Enosawa S, Matsuno N, Kasahara M, Matsunari H, et al. Transgenic pig expressing the red fluorescent protein kusabira-orange as a novel tool for preclinical studies on hepatocyte transplantation. Transplantation Proceedings. 2013;**45**:1808-1810. DOI: 10.1016/j.transproceed.2013.01.017

[60] Takeuchi H, Niki Y, Matsunari H, Umeyama K, Nagashima H, Enomoto H, et al. Temporal changes in cellular repopulation and collagen fibril remodeling and regeneration after allograft anterior cruciate ligament reconstruction: An Experimental Study Using Kusabira-Orange Transgenic Pigs. The American Journal of Sports Medicine. 2016;**44**:2375-2383. DOI: 10.1177/0363546516650881

[61] Susaki EA, Tainaka K, Perrin D, Kishino F, Tawara T, Watanabe TM, et al. Whole-brain imaging with single-cell resolution using chemical cocktails and computational analysis. Cell. 2014;**157**:726-739. DOI: 10.1016/j.cell.2014.03.042

[62] Osada H, Kawatou M, Fujita D, Tabata Y, Minatoya K, Yamashita JK, et al. Therapeutic potential of clinical-grade human induced pluripotent stem cell-derived cardiac tissues. JTCVS Open. 2021;**8**:359-374. DOI: 10.1016/j.xjon.2021.09.038

[63] Ng EW, Wong MY, Poon TC. Advances in MALDI mass spectrometry in clinical diagnostic applications. Topics in Current Chemistry. 2014;**336**:139-175. DOI: 10.1007/128_2012_413

[64] Bassols A, Costa C, Eckersall PD, Osada J, Sabria J, Tibau J. The pig as an animal model for human pathologies: A proteomics perspective. Proteomics. Clinical Applications. 2014;**8**:715-731. DOI: 10.1002/prca.201300099

[65] Linscheid N, Santos A, Poulsen PC, Mills RW, Calloe K, Leurs U, et al.

Quantitative proteome comparison of human hearts with those of model organisms. PLoS Biology. 2021;**19**:e3001144. DOI: 10.1371/journal.pbio.3001144

[66] Tamiyakul H, Kemter E, Kosters M, Ebner S, Blutke A, Klymiuk N, et al. Progressive proteome changes in the myocardium of a pig model for Duchenne muscular dystrophy. iScience. 2020;**23**:101516. DOI: 10.1016/j.isci.2020.101516

[67] Muller T, Boileau E, Talyan S, Kehr D, Varadi K, Busch M, et al. Updated and enhanced pig cardiac transcriptome based on long-read RNA sequencing and proteomics. Journal of Molecular and Cellular Cardiology. 2021;**150**:23-31. DOI: 10.1016/j.yjmcc.2020.10.005

[68] Dubois E, Fertin M, Burdese J, Amouyel P, Bauters C, Pinet F. Cardiovascular proteomics: Translational studies to develop novel biomarkers in heart failure and left ventricular remodeling. Proteomics. Clinical Applications. 2011;**5**:57-66. DOI: 10.1002/prca.201000056

[69] Mandai M, Kurimoto Y, Takahashi M. Autologous induced stem-cell-derived retinal cells for macular degeneration. The New England Journal of Medicine. 2017;**377**:792-793. DOI: 10.1056/NEJMc1706274

[70] Sugita S, Iwasaki Y, Makabe K, Kamao H, Mandai M, Shiina T, et al. Successful transplantation of retinal pigment epithelial cells from MHC homozygote iPSCs in MHC-Matched models. Stem Cell Reports. 2016;**7**:635-648. DOI: 10.1016/j.stemcr.2016.08.010

[71] Morizane A, Kikuchi T, Hayashi T, Mizuma H, Takara S, Doi H, et al. MHC matching improves engraftment of iPSC-derived neurons in non-human primates. Nature Communications. 2017;**8**:385. DOI: 10.1038/s41467-017-00926-5

[72] Li C, Chen S, Zhou Y, Zhao Y, Liu P, Cai J. Application of induced pluripotent stem cell transplants: Autologous or allogeneic? Life Sciences. 2018;**212**:145-149. DOI: 10.1016/j.lfs.2018.09.057

[73] Medicetty S, Wiktor D, Lehman N, Raber A, Popovic ZB, Deans R, et al. Percutaneous adventitial delivery of allogeneic bone marrow-derived stem cells via infarct-related artery improves long-term ventricular function in acute myocardial infarction. Cell Transplantation. 2021;**21**:1109-1120. DOI: 10.3727/096368911X603657

[74] Shiba Y, Gomibuchi T, Seto T, Wada Y, Ichimura H, Tanaka Y, et al. Allogeneic transplantation of iPS cell-derived cardiomyocytes regenerates primate hearts. Nature. 2016;**538**:388-391. DOI: 10.1038/nature19815

[75] Kawamura T, Miyagawa S, Fukushima S, Maeda A, Kashiyama N, Kawamura A, et al. Cardiomyocytes derived from MHC-homozygous induced pluripotent stem cells exhibit reduced allogeneic immunogenicity in MHC-matched non-human primates. Stem Cell Reports. 2016;**6**:312-320. DOI: 10.1016/j.stemcr.2016.01.012

[76] Murata K, Ikegawa M, Minatoya K, Masumoto H. Strategies for immune regulation in iPS cell-based cardiac regenerative medicine. Inflammation Regeneration. 2020;**40**:36. DOI: 10.1186/s41232-020-00145-4

[77] Ando A, Imaeda N, Ohshima S, Miyamoto A, Kaneko N, Takasu M, et al. Characterization of swine leukocyte antigen alleles and haplotypes on a novel miniature pig line, Microminipig. Animal Genetics. 2014;**45**:791-798. DOI: 10.1111/age.12199

[78] Xu J, Yu L, Guo J, Xiang J, Zheng Z, Gao D, et al. Generation of pig induced pluripotent stem cells using an extended pluripotent stem cell culture system. Stem Cell Research & Therapy. 2019;**10**:193. DOI: 10.1186/s13287-019-1303-0

[79] Chakritbudsabong W, Chaiwattanarungruengpaisan S, Sariya L, Pamonsupornvichit S, Ferreira JN, Sukho P, et al. Exogenous LIN28 is required for the maintenance of self-renewal and pluripotency in presumptive porcine-induced pluripotent stem cells. Frontiers in Cell and Development Biology. 2021;**9**:709286. DOI: 10.3389/fcell.2021.709286

[80] Choi KH, Lee DK, Oh JN, Kim SH, Lee M, Woo SH, et al. Pluripotent pig embryonic stem cell lines originating from in vitro-fertilized and parthenogenetic embryos. Stem Cell Research. 2020;**49**:102093. DOI: 10.1016/j.scr.2020.102093

[81] Su Y, Zhu J, Salman S, Tang Y. Induced pluripotent stem cells from farm animals. Journal of Animal Science. Nov 1, 2020;**98**(11):skaa343. DOI: 10.1093/jas/skaa343

[82] Madden JC, Hewitt M, Przybylak K, Vandebriel RJ, Piersma AH, Cronin MT. Strategies for the optimisation of in vivo experiments in accordance with the 3Rs philosophy. Regulatory Toxicology and Pharmacology. 2012;**63**:140-154. DOI: 10.1016/j.yrtph.2012.03.010